I0441838

COVID-19: GOING BEYOND ROUTINE?

SHATHEES BASKARAN

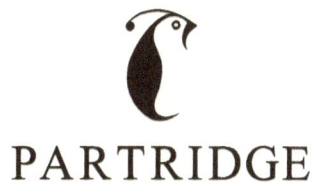

PARTRIDGE

ISBN: Softcover   978-1-5437-6997-5
               eBook   978-1-5437-6998-2

To order additional copies of this book, contact
Toll Free +65 3165 7531 (Singapore)
Toll Free +60 3 3099 4412 (Malaysia)
orders.singapore@partridgepublishing.com

www.partridgepublishing.com/singapore

CONTENTS

DISCLAIMER

The author reserves the right not to be responsible for the topicality, correctness, completeness, or quality of the information provided. Liability claims regarding damage caused by the use of any information provided, including any kind of information which is incomplete or incorrect, will therefore be rejected. All offers are not-binding and without obligation. Parts of the pages or the complete publication including all offers and information might be extended, changed, or partly or completely deleted by the author without a separate announcement. Because of the dynamic nature of the Internet, any web addresses or links contained in this book may have changed since publication and may no longer be valid.

You may not copy, reproduce, distribute, publish, display, perform, modify, create derivative works, transmit, or in any way exploit any such content, nor may you distribute any part of this content over any network, including a local area network, sell or offer it for sale, or use such content to construct any kind of database. Reusing this document is expressly prohibited without prior written permission from the editor and authors.

LIST OF CONTRIBUTORS

Shathees Baskaran *Azman Hashim International Business School, Universiti Teknologi Malaysia, Johor Bahru*

Kesavan Nallaluthan *Faculty of Management & Economics, Universiti Pendidikan Sultan Idris, Perak, Malaysia*

Sethuprakhash Vengidason *Faculty of Technical and Vocational Education, Universiti Pendidikan Sultan Idris, Perak, Malaysia*

Uma Shangery Aruldass *Azman Hashim International Business School, Universiti Teknologi Malaysia, Johor Bahru*

Shatish Rao Samtharam *Azman Hashim International Business School, Universiti Teknologi Malaysia, Johor Bahru*

Priyaa Tharisiny Aruldass *Azman Hashim International Business School, Universiti Teknologi Malaysia, Johor Bahru*

Logaiswari Indiran *Azman Hashim International Business School, Universiti Teknologi Malaysia, Johor Bahru*

Santhi Ramanathan *Faculty of Business, Multimedia University, Melaka*

ABOUT AUTHORS

Dr. Shathees Baskaran has a Bachelor of Economics from Universiti Putra Malaysia, an MBA (Accountancy), and a Doctor of Business Administration from Universiti Utara Malaysia. Shathees Baskaran is an experienced strategic management professional who has worked with some of the world's most respected and recognizable brands for more than 15 years. His major area of teaching and research interests are strategic management, entrepreneurship, and related behavioural studies where his intellectual contributions can be found.

Dr. Kesavan Nallaluthan is a Senior Lecturer at the Faculty of Management and Economics, Sultan Idris Education University, Perak, Malaysia. He has an MBA and a Doctor of Business Administration, and is currently, a full-time academician, who has over 14 years of work experience in manufacturing and the R&D process. His area of interest in teaching and research are entrepreneurship, strategic management, and industrial management.

Dr. Sethuprakhash Vengidason is an Associate Professor at the Faculty of Technical and Vocational, Sultan Idris Education University, Perak, Malaysia. He has a BSc, MSc, and a Doctor of philosophy in chemistry and is currently, a full-time lecturer who has over 17 years of work experience in Lecturing and research work. His area of interest is safety practices and chemistry.

Ms. Uma Shangery Aruldass is an ardent Aerospace fan from Malaysia, a working professional, currently attached to an International Airline in Malaysia. Uma has completed her Bachelor's Degree in Aerospace Engineering and Master's in Aviation Management. She is undertaking her Professional Certification for her research experience in Active Space Debris Removal using CubeSats projects. She has also bagged an International award for 'Outstanding Solution for the Case Study' by International Civil Aviation Organization (ICAO) in 2018 for her case presentation in China.

Mr. Shatish Rao Samtharam has a Bachelor of Management (Operation) from Universiti Sains Malaysia and an MBA (Strategic Management) from Universiti Teknologi Malaysia. Shatish Rao is an experienced professional who has worked with reputable multinational and conglomerate companies for more than 6 years. He has vast experience in analyzing customer behaviours and sustainability development for corporate companies. His main forte is performing critical research studies and analyses in business and management environments.

Ms. Priyaa Tharisiny Aruldass has graduated from Universiti Malaysia Sabah with a Bachelor's Degree in Geology. Later, she spread her wings and obtained a Master's Degree in Business Administration from Universiti Teknologi Malaysia. She has served as a Customer Specialist Executive in Grab Malaysia HQ during the Covid19 breakout era. Currently, she is working in the supply chain department of a Multinational Company based in Penang, Malaysia. She is deeply passionate about public speaking and philanthropic activities.

Dr. Logaiswari Indiran graduated from the University of Malaya with a Bachelor of Business Administration (Hons) and obtained a Master of Education (Technical and Vocational) and a Ph.D. (Management) from the Universiti Teknologi Malaysia.

Currently, she is a faculty at AHIBS specializing in technology entrepreneurship, innovation, intellectual capital, business incubators, and start-ups.

Dr. Santhi Ramanathan, a senior Lecturer, was leading the Economic Unit at the Faculty of Business, Multimedia University, Melaka, Malaysia, where she has been attached for the last 20 years. She has extensive teaching experience, having taught numerous undergraduate modules and supervise post-graduate and research scholars. Dr. Santhi's research interests include Development Economics, Globalisation, and Sustainable Development. She has published several journal articles and book chapters at the national and international levels.

PREFACE

The development of IR 4.0 has become a new direction for all organizations and ecosystems around it to lead the more rapid development towards a business world that is expected to bring a variety of innovations. As a result, many organizations are implementing large-scale transition plans to capitalize on these developments or simply to stay up with rivals as emergent breakthroughs fundamentally restructure the sector. However, it is undeniable that IR 4.0 will take quite a long time to realize the aspirations dreamed of by not only the organization but the entire ecosystem who can't wait to see the glory of innovation to come.

However, the sudden advent of unexpected disruptions, far from the human ability to predict has led to an acceleration of the need to identify, create and implement digital transformations that will be able to fast-track these innovations. In the serenity of doing business, nobody expected a surprise that will shake this world without any sign. It was March 11, 2020, when World Health Organization declared COVID-19 a pandemic. Far from the eye and far beyond the distance, and that's what people thought when the coronavirus started its activities in Wuhan city of mainland China. It does not reach the human mind that the advent of the corona will not only be a threat to health but will also change the way of life and ruin the business empire that has been built for so long.

The arrival of COVID-19 has indeed brought about a tremendous challenge that is difficult to explain in ordinary words. The impact on individuals, organizations whether micro, small, large, or multinational, companies, and ecosystems as a whole is extraordinary. The paralysis of the strength of the household economy, the disruption of the organization's supply chain, the interruption to the country's economic activities, and the strain on the country's healthcare system are a few notable areas. Human ignorance of the power of the corona not only shocked the whole world but also proved to all organizations the weakness of the business model that has existed for so long. Hence, "business as usual" has become a thing of the past, thanks to the coronavirus. This proves that in this unpredictable age, there is no such thing as "normal". Many companies have begun their recovery process as the effects of COVID-19 continue to be felt. However, a pandemic that is continuing to peak with adverse effects on organizational efforts made the business landscape to be much different than it was in the past. To emerge stronger is the only way for organizations to reinvent themselves as they step into and post-pandemic business environment.

In light of the continuing pandemic and uncertainty surrounding the organizations, assumptions historically used to formulate strategic options in setting their strategic path are now being called into question. Altering those presumptions, re-evaluating all circumstances, and progressing their capacity to predict and respond in an opportune way are all part of this process now. Organizations that are capable of navigating uncertainty will be better prepared with the ability to survive through high resilience regardless of any upcoming changes. There is still no sign of when the pandemic that has plagued this world will end. However, the shock that arose over the past year has now become a new norm, and organizations and customers have begun to adjust to this new routine.

Key Characteristics of Future Strategy – Long Known, Less Embraced

COVID-19 has put enormous pressure on businesses today. Its emergence has shown indications that the decisions made today will influence how businesses will be carried out tomorrow. This is not all, but there are many more disruptions to come, and organizations today are required to plan their future with carefully designed business strategies given current organizational circumstances to endure the forthcoming challenges. There are varying views on predicting future strategies by experts across the world. Nevertheless, there are two important determinants in predicting future strategies for an organization. The first is organizational resilience and the second will be organizational agility.

While resilience is a dynamic concept, in general terms organizational resilience refers to the organization's ability to adapt, survive, and return to a "normality" state after the occurrence of unexpected turbulences although there is a general thinking that to be resilient is to bend but not to break. Usually, an organization that has low resilience to exogenous changes and shocks will start to recover from perturbations with its adaptive capacity while starting to innovate to recuperate from the disruptions caused by the environment. However, an organization with rigid structures is less resilient to exogenous changes and shocks since there are no slack resources to adapt to changing business dynamics. A change of rigid structures to a more resilient adaptive capacity requires far-reaching changes, whether innate or deliberate in the business strategy that will be different from the pre-crisis period. This may lead the organizations to fundamentally a different state by creating new ways of doing business. In this sense, strategic resilience which reinvents business models is needed for the success of an organization during business turbulences.

Organizational agility refers to a company's ability to quickly identify and respond to opportunities and challenges. Environmental changes are anticipated by agile organizations, and they act on them as they occur. Because of the turbulence of many areas, such as that caused by rapid environmental, agility is essential. To add to the existing complexities, the changes brought are shifting at a breakneck rate. Any organization, regardless of scale, is fighting to stay competitive and sustainable in the minds of its consumers and community. Customers are more educated than ever before, and they have greater aspirations than they have in the past. In this unpredictably VUCA market, only high-performing, well-adapting, and agility-driven organizations can succeed. This basic premise reveals the significant change in perspective that agile companies need for them to face economic shocks and subsequent changes in market characteristics and consumer behaviours. An adaptable and long-lasting story that connects and leads organizations through the unknown future. An operational model that boosts the company's adaptability and responsiveness across the board recognizes that an organization is in a dynamic adaptive environment in which everyone is responsible for embracing agility continually.

Combinations of these dimensions (whether high or low) will lead to alternative future scenarios for organizations. These two dimensions will also enable the organizations to position their organizations based on their current circumstances and then to determine the scenarios of the future and ultimately design alternative future business strategies which are expected to be impactful and enhance their business continuity and sustainability.

What's Next?

The emergence of IR 4.0 and its acceleration through the coronavirus's appearance allows everyone to reconsider the changes we've to embrace in our lives and businesses. The modern world requires a stronger, but more robust architecture that addresses both global challenges and opportunities. The overall challenges in the industry thrown by IR4.0 are still not fully addressed, and covid-19 arrives with another very strong impact, making the present state more uncontrollable. COVID-19 was a visible contributor to the market collapse of 2020 without any sign of near future rebound, and the economies were still vulnerable and precarious. The pain and uncertainty of market crashes are continuing and it is unclear if this is normal in a "new normal" business environment. If so, uncertainties whether the industries are ready for (further) market consolidations as a result of financial collapses, will micro, small, and medium enterprises make a comeback or worse will be forced to exit and re-enter the market with a fresh yet different business model are still surrounded by countless assumptions. It is essential to acknowledge that COVID-19's effect would be strongly influenced by how long the pandemic lasts. By the time the global pandemic comes to an end which remained uncertain, most of the economic chains will be disrupted, collapsing small boys and forcing them to exit the economic system, weakening the big boys forcing them to either undergo rescaling or to a worse extent, to exit the market, and stronger boys take control through consolidation. Moreover, if the situation is expected to get worse, are they prepared for the next crash? What will this lead to, especially in the context of market consolidation and restructuring? Where is the fate of small traders who are no longer able to survive due to further market crashes which are still ambiguous? This leads to viewing the future from three different focus areas, namely the new (consolidated) markets, the customers defined by these new markets, and also the organizational strategies driven by re-segmented consumer characteristics.

Consumer characteristics are an all-time significant component in a business architecture since a greater understanding of consumer preferences and experiences will greatly assist an organization to perform and more importantly be competitive and stay relevant in the marketplace. The rapid development in technology in IR 4.0 and internet technology has had a significant effect on how people collaborate, interact, and perform business practices. To add to this severity, the emergence of coronavirus has not accelerated the pace but also has reshaped the customers' and consumers characteristics. Changes in the world have inevitably resulted in the introduction of new customer and marketplace perspectives. Unimaginable changes brought about by coronavirus coupled with pacing IR 4.0 have shown that consumers are transforming into active users of an online lifestyle that has significantly accelerated their shopping journey by allowing complete flexibility to their choices and decisions. The drastic turnaround in customers' and consumers' lifestyles has questioned traditional practices of understanding them, instead of calling for identification and classification of technology-defined consumer characteristics. This is set as the second most focus in resigning the business strategy. The successful adoption of a digital lifestyle eliminates the geographical radius of their options and possibly removes the stickiness of dedicated merchants. Owing to multiple borderless options, customers will start moving virtually beyond their geographical location, keeping aside the spatial distance to optimize their seamless customer experience, prompting the further proliferation of limitless niche market segments and consequently splintering share of wallet across many providers.

Given that the time taken to gain global public immunity is limited, the first focus portrays a scenario in which organizations resume routine operations after a reasonable recovery from the period of downturn. This recovery may no longer follow traditional business models. I shift in business models is an unavoidable imperative for organizations. As market consolidation is underway, the emerging market structures will redefine the newer characteristics of the value-conscious consumers. The traditional approaches such as loyalty programs may require new ways of creating their raving fans and certainly will disrupt current practices in place requiring remodelling of their value prepositions. In a consolidated market structure, commonly accepted value prepositions (operational excellence, product leadership, or customer intimacy) may remain valid but what alterations are needed will be dictated by the re-segmentation of the organizations' relevant market. Given changes in the marketplace and its governing structures, a redefinition of customer trustworthiness, customer satisfaction, and customer referrals may pose newer challenges to organizations' sustainability. What is more important for the organization will be to embrace a drastic change in its strategy, processes, and mindset from a business strategy supported by technology to technology-led business strategies.

Shathees Baskaran
Azman Hashim International Business School
Universiti Teknologi Malaysia
2022

CHAPTER 1

COVID-19 and Plausible Organizational Scenarios

Shathees Baskaran

1.1 INTRODUCTION

The world has recorded multiple significant pandemics which have resulted in severe consequences for various stakeholders. One such kind is an outbreak of infectious diseases that had cross-border implications and threatened and collapsed economies (Verikios, Sullivan, Stojanovski, Giesecke, & Woo, 2015; Davies, 2013; Drake, Chalabi, & Coker, 2012). Once

1

again, the world has recorded another pandemic, COVID-19, presenting debilitating challenges to organizations and nations across the world. Organizations have witnessed a serious impact when the COVID-19 crisis struck and more importantly, these organizations have become vulnerable to their uncertain long-term sustainability. This, in turn, has forced the organizations to consider new normal of doing business by considering the potential impact of this pandemic. This review is aimed to readdress two very prominent organizational characteristics, namely resilience, and agility in anticipating unforeseen business challenges. An assessment of these characteristics will suggest a four-quadrant matrix portraying plausible organizational scenarios depending on their current level of resiliency and agility in the organization. Next, a discussion will follow about the new normal business model in response to organizational challenges and the organization of the book.

1.2 ORGANIZATIONAL CHARACTERISTICS

COVID-19 has put enormous pressure on businesses today. Its emergence has shown indications that the decisions made today will influence how businesses will be carried out tomorrow. This is not all, but there are many more disruptions to come, and organizations today are required to plan their future with carefully designed business strategies given current organizational circumstances to endure the forthcoming challenges. There are varying views on predicting future strategies by experts across the world. Nevertheless, there are two important determinants in predicting future strategies for an organization. The first is organizational resilience and the second will be organizational agility. Combinations of these dimensions (whether high or low) will lead to alternative future scenarios for an organization. These two dimensions will also enable the organizations to position their organizations based on their current circumstances and then to determine the scenarios of the future and ultimately design alternative future business strategies which are expected to be impactful and enhance their business continuity and sustainability. Although both agility and resilience are important dimensions, it exists only when there is a presence of organizational slack as it provides important spare resources to be used in critical times. An organization with spare resources will allow the organizational members to enjoy additional resources that are needed to take a forward-looking perspective beyond current business while exploring emerging opportunities (to be capitalized) and threats (to be overcome). On the other hand, the existence of organizational slack improves the resilience of the organization. The availability of slack resources allows faster redeployment of these resources in response to unexpected shocks so that the organization can be repaired quickly and resume its operations without continuous suffering. Nevertheless, an organization that is flawlessly designed indicates a strong organizational and strategic fit hence the availability of organizational slack could be a real challenge. Therefore, organizations need to check if their current organizational configurations are allowing the allocation of adequate organizational slack in enabling agility and resilience. Accounting for versatility in organizational slack in organizational systems and structure will ensure quick adaptability to foreseen and unforeseen external forces, hence ensuring the continued business operation of the organization with minimal disruptions. The following sections will provide a detailed discussion about organizational resilience and organizational agility.

1.2.1 Organizational Resilience

Inevitable business disruptions have made "resilience" gain increasing attention from scholars as well as practitioners. This term originated from a Latin word called "resiliere," which means to "bounce back". The Literature has shown definitions as shown in Table 1.1:

Table 1.1 Definitions of Resilience

Author	Definition
Walker (2013)	The capacity of a system to absorb disturbance, re-organize, and keep functioning in much the same way as before
Kindra (2013)	The ability of a system, community, or society exposed to hazards to resist, absorb, accommodate and recover from the effects of a hazard in a timely and efficient manner
Barthel and Isendahl (2013)	The capacity to absorb shocks, utilize them, re-organize, and continue to develop without losing fundamental functions
Boto et al. (2013)	The ability of critical physical infrastructure to absorb shocks... is the process of adaptation and of developing a set of skills, capacities, behaviours, and actions necessary when dealing with adversity
Anderies et al. (2013)	The capacity to sustain a shock and continue to function and, more generally, cope with change

Author	Definition
Bahadur et al. (2013)	The continued ability of a person, group, or system to adapt to stress – such, as any sort of disturbance – so that it may continue to function, or quickly recover its ability to function, during and after stress
Béné et al. (2012)	Not just about the ability to maintain or return to a previous state; it is about adapting and learning to live with changes and uncertainty
Mitchell and Harris (2012)	The ability of a system and its parts to anticipate, absorb, accommodate, or recover from the effects of a shock or stress in a timely and efficient manner
Gitz & Meybeck (2012)	The ability of a system and its parts to anticipate, absorb, accommodate or recover from the effects of a hazardous event in a timely and efficient manner, including by ensuring the preservation, restoration, or improvement of its essential basic structures and functions
Mitchell & Harris (2012)	The ability of a substance or object to spring back into shape; the capacity to recover quickly from difficulties
Frankenberger et al. (2012)	The ability of countries, communities, and households to efficiently anticipate, adapt to, and/or recover from the effects of potentially hazardous occurrences (natural disasters, economic instability, and conflict) in a manner that protects livelihoods, accelerates, and sustains recovery, and supports economic growth.

Author	Definition
Pain & Levine (2012)	The capacity of people or "systems" to cope with stresses and shocks by anticipating them, preparing for them, responding to them, and recovering from them
Moberg and Simonsen (2011)	The capacity of a system, be it an individual, a forest, a city, or an economy, to deal with change and continue to develop
Montalbano (2011)	The capacity of a system, community, or society potentially exposed to hazards to adapt, by resisting or changing to reach and maintain an acceptable level of functioning and structure
Pregenzer (2011)	The measure of a system's ability to absorb continuous and unpredictable change and still maintain its vital functions
Vugrin et al. (2010)	Given the occurrence of a particular disruptive event (or set of events), the resilience of a system to that event (or events) is that system's ability to reduce efficiently both the magnitude and duration of deviation from targeted system performance levels
Otobi (2010)	A multi-dimensional construct is defined as the capacity of individuals, families, communities, and institutions to anticipate, withstand, and/or judiciously engage with a catastrophic event and/or experience; actively making meaning out of adversity, to maintain normal functions without losing identity

Author	Definition
Cadman et al. (2010)	The capacity of an ecosystem to absorb change and re-organize itself, whilst changing, to retain its character and ecological functioning
Haimes (2009)	The ability of the system to withstand a major disruption within acceptable degradation parameters and to recover with a suitable time and reasonable costs and risks
Oxfam (2009)	The ability of a joint social and ecological system – such as a farm – to withstand shocks, coupled with the capacity to learn from them and evolve in response to changing conditions
Badahur (2009)	The capacity of a system to anticipate, prepare for, respond to and quickly recover from changes in the system – be it climate shock and stresses or other drivers of change
Bapna et al. (2009)	The ability to handle stresses or recover from disturbances or shocks. In the most positive sense, it is the capacity to thrive in the face of challenges. Resilience in the context of rural resource-dependent communities is comprised of ecological resilience, social resilience, and economic resilience
Boyd et al. (2008)	A system's capacity to deal with change and to continue to develop
Cumming et al. (2005)	The ability of the system to maintain its identity in the face of internal change and external shocks and disturbances

7

Author	Definition
Walker et al. (2004)	The capacity to absorb disturbance and reorganize while changing to still retain essentially the same function, structure, identity, and feedback
Allenby and Fink (2000)	The capability of the system to maintain its function and structure against internal and external changes and downgrade the performance of the system when it must.
Carter & May (2001)	The ability of the household to recover from the shock.
Barnett (2001)	The capacity to cope with uncertainty and surprises while maintaining overall system persistence… resilience is about learning from error how to bounce back in better shape
Holling (1973)	The measure of the persistence of systems and of their ability to absorb change and disturbance and still maintain the same relationships between populations or state variables

While resilience is a dynamic concept, in general terms organizational resilience refers to the organization's ability to adapt, survive, and return to a "normality" state after the occurrence of unexpected turbulences although there is a general thinking that to be resilient is to bend but not to break. Usually, an organization that has low resilience to exogenous changes and shocks will start to recover from perturbations with its adaptive capacity while starting to innovate to recuperate from the disruptions caused by the environment. However, an organization with rigid structures is less resilient to exogenous changes and shocks since there are no slack resources to adapt to changing business dynamics. A change of rigid structures to a more resilient adaptive capacity requires far-reaching changes, whether innate or deliberate in the business strategy that will be different than the pre-crisis period. This may lead the organizations to fundamentally a different state by creating new ways of doing business. In this sense, strategic resilience which reinvents business models is needed for the success of an organization during business turbulences.

1.2.2 Organizational Agility

The world is evolving at a breakneck pace. This evolvement needs the organization to stay relevant in the eyes of its customers, society, and stakeholders. Because of the increasing changes in many situations, agility has become essential. The capacity of a company to recognize and respond to opportunities and dangers quickly and effectively is referred to as organizational agility. Simply said, business agility is an organization's ability and desire to adapt to, generate, and utilize change for the benefit of its customers. Hence, environmental shifts are anticipated by agile organizations, and they respond to them as they occur. This indicates an operational approach that boosts the organization's agility and responsiveness across the board to remain relevant and sustainable. A multitude of definitions are shown in the literature as displayed in Table 1.2:

Table 1.2 Definitions of Agility

Author	Definition
Ross (2008)	The use of existing IT and business process capabilities to rapidly generate new business value while limiting costs and risks.

Author	Definition
Mathiyakalan et al. (2005)	The ability of an organization to detect changes (which can be opportunities or threats or a combination of both) in its business environment and hence provide focused and rapid response to its customers and stakeholders by reconfiguring its resources, processes, and strategies
Raschke and David (2005)	The ability of a firm to dynamically modify and/or reconfigure individual business processes to accommodate the required and potential needs of the firm
Ashrafi et al. (2005)	An organization's ability to sense environmental changes and respond effectively and efficiently to that change
Sambamurthy and Zmud (2004)	The ability of a firm to continually sense and explore customer and marketplace enrichment opportunities and respond with the appropriate configurations of capabilities and capacities to exploit these opportunities with speed, surprise, and competitive success.
Conboy and Fitzgerald (2004)	The continual readiness of an entity to rapidly or inherently, proactively or reactively, embrace change, through high quality, simplistic, economical components and relationships with its environment.

Author	Definition
Sambamurthy et al. (2003)	The ability of a firm to redesign its existing processes rapidly and create new processes in a timely fashion to be able to take advantage of and thrive in the unpredictable and highly dynamic market conditions
Menor et al. (2001)	The ability of a firm to excel simultaneously on operations capabilities of quality, delivery, flexibility, and cost in a coordinated fashion
Dove (2001)	The ability of an organization to respond efficiently and effectively to both proactive and reactive needs and opportunities in the ace of an unpredictable and uncertain environment
Hooper et al (2001)	The ability of an enterprise to develop and exploit its inter-and intra-organizational capabilities.
Ramasesh et al (2001)	The successful exploration of competitive bases (speed, flexibility, innovation pro-activity, quality, and profitability) through the integration of reconfigurable resources, and best practices in a knowledge-rich environment to provide customer-driven products and services in a fast-changing market environment.
Zhang & Sharifi (2000)	The ability of enterprises to cope with unexpected changes, survive unprecedented threats from the business environment, and take advantage of changes as opportunities.

Author	Definition
Yusuf et al. (1999)	Successful exploration of competitive bases (speed, flexibility, innovation, proactivity, quality, and profitability) through the integration of reconfigurable resources and knowledge management to provide customer-driven products and services in a fast-changing market environment
Fliedner and Vokurka (1997)	Ability to market successfully low-cost, high-quality products with short lead times and in varying volumes that provide enhanced value to customers through customization
Cho et al. (1996)	Capability to survive and prosper in a competitive environment or continuous and unpredictable changes by reacting quickly and effectively to changing markets, designed by customer-designed products and services
Kumar and Motwani (1995)	Ability to accelerate the activities on the critical path and time-based competitiveness
Goldman et al. (1995)	The capability of an organization to operate profitability in a competitive environment comprised of continually changing customer habits

Author	Definition
Goldman et al., (1995)	The ability to thrive in a competitive environment of continuous and unanticipated change and to respond quickly to rapidly changing, fragmenting global markets that are served by networked competitors with routine access to a worldwide production system and are driven by demand for high-quality, high-performance, low-cost, customer-configured products and services.
D'Aveni (1994)	The ability to detect opportunities for innovation and seize those competitive market opportunities by assembling requisite assets, knowledge, and relationships with speed and surprise.

Various definitions of agility infer that a change, unforeseen and unexpected, speed and rapidity, reconfigurable and adaptable, monitoring and sensing, pro-active and reactive reaction, innovation, learning, inter-and intra-organizational skills are some of the concepts used to define business agility. Agility is fluid, open-ended, and context-dependent (in time and space).

Agility is critical for all businesses, but it is especially critical for organizations in fast-changing environments. There are many reasons which highlight the need for agility. To begin with, an organization is well-positioned to move faster and more efficiently by adjusting itself to defy its competitors in the quickest time possible. Next, an agile organization can leap ahead of its rivals by making quick strategic moves allowing an adaption to environmental changes. Finally, being more agile than rivals can, in certain cases, be a competitive advantage in and of itself, in addition to being a weapon for countering strategic actions by competitors or gaining a competitive advantage. This rising need for agility has sparked a competition for better agility, with the losers potentially paying a high price.

1.3 PLAUSIBLE ORGANIZATIONAL SCENARIOS

Organizations in a competitive environment face rapid changes in their surroundings. In this vein, resilience and agility are becoming important pillars for an organization's sustainability. This is because it increases readiness, robustness, and flexibility in uncertain environments. Additionally, it allows the organizations to deal with and mitigate disruption, as well as predict its incidence and consequences through efficient assessment of risk, effective allocation, and mobilization of resources leading to timely decision-making by expanding access to a wide range of solutions to specific issues.

Four distinctive typologies are proposed in explaining the level of resilience and agility among the organizations, namely Preserve (being the most resilient and agile), Revive (being resilient but less agile), Renew (being agile but less resilient), and Exit (being the least resilient and agile) as shown in Figure 1.1 below:

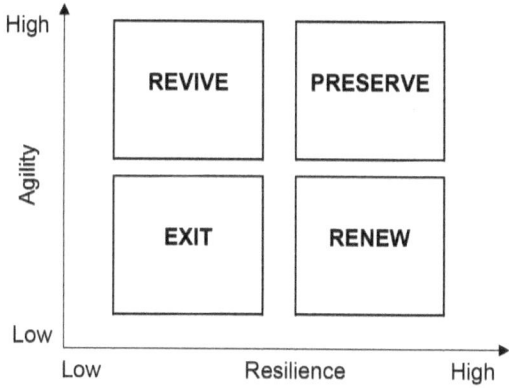

Figure 1.1 Resilience-Agility Business Scenario Matrix

1.3.1 Scenario 1: Preserve

The first typology, "Preserve" depicts organizations that are very agile and resilient in their operating model. The business model is very fluid to accommodate and pro-act to the forthcoming challenges. Organizations that fall within this typology are quick to return to normal operation after a very short recessionary period. Usually, they are well-positioned to flatten the impact of the unexpected environmental forces to continue to survive and kick start the next curve of growth. Ultimately, this is the ideal situation, and it is something all organizations strive for. Companies, on the other hand, may experience revenue shocks as a result of various disruptions in their operational activities, but they may persevere and survive-thanks to the relatively short time it takes to develop immunity to environmental shocks, allowing organizations to return to a normal state with sufficient resilience and agility. The organization that falls within this typology is found to employ what Wenzel, Stanske, and Lieberman (2020) call the enduring business approach in a crisis like this to discover solutions to keep their operations running as usual during the crisis.

1.3.2 Scenario 2: Renew

The second typology called "Renew" depicts organizations that are very resilient in their operation although these types of organizations are not necessarily agile. Its resilience can be contributed by various factors including financial strength to manage the disruptions. Organizations falling into this typology can withstand the disruptions to their business model. These organizations can adapt, survive longer, and return to "normality" after facing unexpected turbulences although they are slow in tackling the disruptions. Despite this resilience, the organizations are slow and ineffective in tackling environmental issues due to the lower level of agility. This may lead the organizations to adopt a retrenchment strategy to remain in the business (Wenzel et al., 2020) while adapting themselves to the needs of the new operating environment. To remain resilient, tactics such as downsizing and cost reductions will be opted by these organizations to keep the firm afloat amid the long-term economic downturn. This strategy allows the organizations to endure for extended periods until their business returns to a normal state.

1.3.3 Scenario 3: Revive

The third typology is known as "Revive". Organizations in Revive typology tend to be more agile with a lower level of resilience. These types of organizations are normally very quick in tackling disruptions. Given the lower resilience, these organizations will try to adapt to the new environment by embracing a downsizing strategy, for example. Usually, driven by stronger agility, these types of organizations innovate by reallocating resources to a newer business model. These organizations aim to stay in the business by taking necessary measures although it may lead to resizing of the organization. Organizations are no longer allowed to operate in the same manner as before hence a new normal will emerge as a result of this scenario. Organizations within this typology will adopt innovative strategies as it will be the most appropriate (Wenzel et al., 2020) to move in line with a higher level of agility which also suffers lower resilience. These will become crucial components of a new business model during this period.

1.3.4 Scenario 4: Exit

The last typology is called "Exit". This scenario depicts a chaotic world in which environmental shock immunity takes a long time to develop and many businesses struggle to stay afloat as the economy becomes overwhelmed. These types of organizations are characterized by lower resilience and agility. This is a situation that all organizations would want to avoid as much as possible. This organization struggles in uncertain environments and is unable to maintain its position in its relevant market. This leads to a massive slowdown in their recovery due to widespread challenges and eventually forces them to adopt an exit strategy to reduce further losses (Wenzel et al., 2020). Nevertheless, organizations may consider innovative strategic moves by reassigning the resources to initiate a new business model consistent with the present demands.

1.4 THE NEW NORMAL BUSINESS MODEL

The novel Coronavirus (COVID-19) pandemic outbreak has thrown a new puzzle to be fixed by not only the healthcare industry and its associated professionals but everyone across the globe in every nation including the business world and also the general public. Coming as a sudden surprise affecting almost every sector in the marketplace, today it has transformed into a worldwide concern. Its velocity of spread has put everyone in awe and challenged the current business models of the organizations, expecting a rapid response to challenges surrounding these organizations. It has created disruptions to existing supply chains while confronting and antagonizing the means and ways of an organization's operations. The pandemic invited or rather challenged the organizations to think, introduce, and execute radical and vigorous approaches to continuing the business operations for its long-term sustainability.

An unexpected COVID-19 episode has surrounded the organizations with a vast number of unknown uncertainties. These obscure dynamics have disrupted organizations across the globe in many ways. In an interlinked business environment, it has disrupted the domestic and international supply chains and eventually has created an unimaginable impact on the continuity of its operations in particular, and its contribution to the national economic development agenda at large. The magnitude of impact as a result of this pandemic reaches greater severity when the business has been compelled to downsize or close during the pandemic. Local and international economic chains are disrupted and forced to change their behavior. By the time the global pandemic comes to an end which is remained uncertain, most of the economic chains will be disrupted, collapsing small boys and forcing them to exit the economic system, weakening the big boys forcing them to either undergo rescaling or to a worse extent, to exit the market, and stronger boys take control through consolidation.

On dubious occasions such as these, plans must be in place to proceed with tasks through crisis circumstances for a speedy resumption of business operations. While a business model is a long-practiced approach, to what extent such approaches are aiding organizations in overcoming a pandemic phobia and its short (to probably mid-term) transitory interruptions is debatable for the subtle attention and relaxed thoughtfulness which may be in existence for the business world to react fast, if not proactively to uncertain episodes affecting the business.

Today, organizations are forced to think not only outside the box but beyond, to discover and consider value-creating business processes that in the past were deemed to be unthinkable or unattainable. Prolonged outbreaks with massive penetration across the globe invited every organization, public, and private to assess their readiness for the potential effect it might have on their business operations and eventual impact on their long-term sustainability.

The focus now has been turned towards restoration and recommence of their business operations to minimize the economic impact to the shareholders, stakeholders, and its economic wellbeing. This has called for a new normal in the business environment. Areas that have remained grey in the past have started to gain more attention and these grey areas have started to visualize greater clarities in doing business differently. It is vigilance and readiness, but not panic behavior that is the most ideal approach to relieve the dangers presented by a COVID-19 pandemic.

Certainly, the pandemic has damaged the current economic model and restated beliefs that exist in economic theories. The long-standing economic principles have been challenged and proven to be not up-to-date. The COVID-19 pandemic has changed the business scene by challenging the business practices and processes installed in place today.

It has provided enough evidence and visibility that tomorrow's condition will be unique, and will present new opportunities to the people who are well prepared while creating disruptions beyond one's imagination to relaxed-minded communities. It is an undeniable truth that the present pandemic and its severe implication for the world are different compared to the disruptions the world has seen and witnessed in the past.

The world is undergoing another cycle of economic challenges. However, the challenges observed in the present COVID-19 crisis are different ball games, insisting the organizations reinvent and redesign their business models towards a new normal.

The normal of today has proven to be less elastic to cater to newer disruptions and there is an inevitable need to look into the new normal of business operations to create a sophisticated, more vigilant, and agile business model to cope with the challenges to be presented in the future. It will be driven by a new regulatory framework across the globe and a very different competitive landscape of industries.

The new, unanticipated challenges posed to the business world have critical implications and need deliberate attention. Many questions are on the list to be addressed. Among others, organizations are facing pressing challenges in redefining the work structure, communication structure, job roles and responsibilities beyond the traditional office atmosphere, triggers and procedures in executing a new normal business model, and the types of tools, technologies, and platforms for a seamless work environment. The COVID-19 pandemic has challenged this self-claimed innovation which was seen as a new way forward as a result of industrial-revolution 4.0. One cannot deny the benefits of this new work structure but the present COVID-19 scenario has proven and very likely, the post-COVID-19 situation will prove that the current structure in place is inadequate and impose new requirements to discover more radical ways for the future business environment.

The new business models as a result of new normal business operations will also have newfangled implications for two important constituents to any business model, namely the business itself and the people being the driver of the business models. The modern world requires a more powerful, yet more robust structure that handles both global threats and possibilities.

1.5 GOING BEYOND THE ROUTINE

The COVID-19 recession has wreaked havoc on certain industries, particularly those that rely on the mobility of people, while leaving others, such as those that rely on the transfer of information, largely unharmed. It has wreaked havoc on industries depending on the movement of people especially and devastated these industries and business sectors. COVID-19 has put them to the test of resilience and agility. This has called for a sharp increase in the attention paid to the existing business model, strategies, processes as well as practices. Multiple concerns and considerations are at play for these industries to restore business sustainability by looking at more radical approaches to preserving their businesses. The following chapters are related to an in-depth exploration of the effect of COVID-19 leading to discussions within the scope of sustainability among some selected industries and areas of concern.

The next chapter discusses the manufacturing industry. The manufacturing industry has been the backbone of the Malaysian economy for many years. The big challenges faced by the manufacturing sectors are the impact on the labor force due to movement control, supply chain disruptions, productivity, etc., due to the COVID-19 pandemic. Industry

4.0 aims to integrate automation and robotics into the seams of a manufacturing base which reduces human error and allows companies to refocus their efforts on areas that generate revenue. Malaysia's economy is facing a tough moment due to the current COVID-19 pandemic. Many manufacturing-related businesses are implementing Industry 4.0 elements to enhance products and processes. This strategy allows businesses that produce and manufacture goods daily to relax a bit on their transactional and financial issues, improving performance, increasing sales, and the relaxation of workers.

The third chapter discusses the view of the covid-19 pandemic towards the airline industry. It explains the impact and situation in an alarming state. The chapter illustrates the cry of the industry and the steps that need to be considered to protect the industry. The impact is viding from system management, people management, and also aircraft management. The chapter explains in-depth the actions that need to be taken for the industry to meet the skies again. The world has seen 'cleaner' skies during the pandemic, which has been a challenge for the airline industry to revive by giving importance to sustainability. Together we stand, to fight the battle by negotiating, advancing, leveraging on the existing resources, and most importantly, by adopting and adapting to the future.

The fourth chapter discusses worldwide lockdowns that have accelerated Work-From-Home (WFH) concept. The chapter revolves around the hard jump-start experienced by the organizations to implement WFH practices during lockdowns. It further discusses the faith in the existing physical work environments and how will they be managed to form a healthier workplace in the future. Besides, work-life boundary management is expected to change due to WFH practices and rapidly evolving technologies. Thus, this chapter upholds work-life integration as an ideal way for employees to manage their work-life demands while working from home. Considering all the changes, WFH will no longer be viewed as a solution during the pandemic, but in a way, it is expected to stay and become a part of organizations for the long run.

The fifth chapter dissects the impacts, both adverse impacts and positive impacts of the covid-19 pandemic on the e-hailing sector. The spinning wheels came to a slow down during the early period of the pandemic. The industry saw a hit in terms of a major drop in car riding bookings, increased operating costs, and a sudden spike in e-hailing platform abuse cases by customers. However, being declared one of the essential services, the e-hailing industry quickly identified many opportunities to stay afloat. One of the golden opportunities that arose was the increase in market demand for online-based food or goods delivery services. The pandemic has been a great challenge and a huge game-changer for the e-hailing industry. The market players try their best to stay afloat by seizing every available opportunity and managing the risks present to cause minimum impact which will be discussed in length in this chapter.

The sixth chapter discusses the unquestionable impact the Covid-19 pandemic has on the global economy and environmental conditions. Small and Medium Enterprises (SMEs), particularly in developing countries, have been hard hit by the Covid-19 outbreak, owing to their limited access to and use of digital technologies. This chapter draws on a review of the literature as well as personal experience to provide assistance to SMEs that are affected by the COVID-19 pandemic. Small and Medium Enterprises (SMEs) are the primary drivers of economic development in Malaysia, where they account for more than 90 percent of all economic activities. They are, however, the most vulnerable to the effects of covid-19, whether from the standpoint of financial risk, digital divide or changed customer behavior, among other factors. This study suggests that future directions toward sustainable practices should be focused on strengthening sustainable development policies, developing sustainable digital infrastructure, and enhancing digital literacy and connectional intelligence.

The final chapter discusses organizational flexibility and the objective approach to explain organizational flexibility that needs continuous exploration to change the principles that set the flexible framework for the organizations to follow and implement. Consequently, the chapter introduces a COVID Business Matrix (known as CoBuM), discussing four characteristics namely Products and Services, Channel, Infrastructure, and Skill in designing post-COVID-19, new normal business strategies in response to COVID-19 challenges.

1.6 CONCLUSION

Many important pandemics have occurred throughout human history, and pandemic-related crises have had tremendous detrimental effects on global health, the economy, and society. Nevertheless, the consequences of a pandemic are severe. One of the prominent consequences is economic instability. Economic losses can cause economic instability due to immediate, long-term, and indirect expenses. In addition, it has also caused social impacts including the closure of social institutions, activities, and events. There are some key issues highlighted by these pandemics which touch on the ability of the organizations to remain sustainable in a crisis. Industries' resilience and agility are very important not only for their sustainability but also to continue to contribute to the economy and nation development. This business does not only become a major contributor to national income but it also associates very closely with United Nations' sustainable development goal 8, "Decent Work and Economic Growth". This highlights its indirect importance and implications for many other facets of business including employment, the standard of living, and also decent lifestyle. Indeed, the sustainability of businesses is a global issue for decades, and today it has received increased attention due to disruptions created by COVID-19. As a result, these firms' sustainability concerns must be carefully addressed for the industry to continue to thrive and have beneficial effects on national economic, and social growth, directly or indirectly. An effective and efficient response to economic shocks can reduce the impact. To ensure that the businesses remain sustainable, business model transformation remains its constant focus to adapt to the dynamic business environment. COVID-19 has steered a paradigm shift in how organizations would approach and adapt their business model in the future as they cope with daily operations in meeting the demands.

ACKNOWLEDGEMENT

Writing a book is harder than I thought and more rewarding than I could have ever imagined. None of this would have been possible without motivation and encouragement from my family, friends, and everyone who was involved directly or indirectly by contributing ideas and perspectives. Finally, my sincere appreciation to all those who have been a part of my getting there.

REFERENCES

Allenby, B., & Fink, J. (2000). Social and ecological resilience: Toward inherently secure and resilient societies. Science, 24(3), 347-64.

Anderies, J.M., Folke, C., Walker, B. & Ostrom, E. (2013). Aligning key concepts for global change policy: robustness, resilience, and sustainability. Ecology and Society 18(2): 8.

Ashrafi, N., Xu, P., Sathasivam, M., Kuilboer, J.P. & Koehler, W. (2005). A Framework for Implementing Business Agility through Knowledge Management Systems. Proceedings of the 2005 Seventh IEEE International Conference on E-Commerce Technology Workshops (CECW'05), pp. 116-121.

Bahadur, A., Ibrahim, M., & Tanner, T. (2013). Characterising Resilience: Unpacking the concept for tackling climate change and development. Climate and Development. 5(1), pp.55-65.

Barnett, J. (2001). Adapting to climate change in Pacific island countries: the problem of uncertainty. World Development, 29, pp. 977-993.

Barthel, S., & Isendahl, C. (2013). Urban gardens, agriculture, and water management: Sources of resilience for long-term food security in cities. Ecol Econ 86:224-234.

Béné, C., Godfrey-Wood, R., Newsham, A. & Davies, M. (2012). Resilience: New utopia or new tyranny? Reflection about the potentials and limits of the concept of resilience in relation to vulnerability reduction programmes. IDS working Paper 405, Brighton: Institute of Development Studies, 61p.

Boyd, E., Osbahr, H., Ericksen, P.J., Tompkins, E.L., Lemos, M.C., & Miller. F. (2008). Resilience and "climatizing" development: examples and policy implications. Development 51, pp. 390-396.

Cadman, M., Petersen, C., Driver, A., Sekhran, N., Maze, K., & Munzhedzi, S. (2010). Biodiversity for Development: South Africa's landscape approach to conserving biodiversity and promoting ecosystem resilience, Pretoria, South Africa: South African National Biodiversity Institute. Available at: https:// cmsdata.iucn.org/ downloads/ primer_11_2_ mb.pdf.

Carter, M.R. & May, J. (2001). One Kind of Freedom: Poverty Dynamics in Post-apartheid South Africa. World Development 29(12), pp. 1987-2006.

Cho, H., Jung, M., Kim, M. (1996). Enabling Technologies of Agile Manufacturing and Its Related Activities in Korea. Comp. Ind. Eng., 30(3), pp. 323-335.

Conboy, K. & Fitzgerald, B. (2004). Toward a conceptual framework of agile methods: a study of agility in different disciplines. Proceedings of the 2004 ACM workshop on Interdisciplinary software engineering research. ACM Press, New York USA.

D'Aveni, R.A. (1994). Hypercompetition: Managing the Dynamics of Strategic Maneuvering. Free Press: NewYork.

Davies, S. E. (2013). National Security and Pandemics. UN Chronicle, 50(2), 20-24.

Dove, R. (2001). Response ability: The language, structure, and culture of the agile enterprise. Hoboken, NJ: John Wiley & Sons.

Drake, T. L., Chalabi, Z., & Coker, R. (2012). Cost-effectiveness analysis of pandemic influenza preparedness: what's missing? Bull World Health Organ, 90(12), 940-941.

Fliedner, G. & Vokurka, R.J. (1997). Agility: competitive weapon of the 1990s and beyond? Production and Inventory Management Journal, 38(3), p.19.

Frankenberger T., Spangler T., Nelson S. and Langworthy M. (2012), Enhancing resilience to food insecurity amid protracted crisis. Paper presented at a High Level Expert Forum on Food Insecurity in Protracted Crises, August 17, 2012. Food and Agriculture Organization, Rome, Italy.

Gitz, V., & Meybeck, A. (2012). Risks, vulnerabilities and resilience in a context of climate change. In Building Resilience for Adaptation to Climate Change in the Agriculture Sector. FAO: Rome, Italy, 23, p. 19.

Goldman, S.L., Nagel, R.N., & Preiss, K. (1995). Agile Competitors andVirtual Organizations: Strategies for

Enriching the Customer. VanNostrand Reinhold, New York.

Haimes, Y.Y. (2009). On the definition of resilience in systems. Risk Analysis, 29(4), 498-501.

Holling, C.S. (1973). Resilience and stability of ecological systems. Annual Review of Ecological Systems, 4, pp. 1-23.

Hooper, M.J., Steeple, D. & Winters, C.N. (2001). Costing customer value: an approach for the agile enterprise. International Journal of Operations and Production Management, 21(5/6), pp. 630-644.

Kindra, J. (2013.) Giving communities a voice in resilience. IRIN Humanitarian News and Analysis. Retrieved from http://www.irinnews.org/report/97595/giving-communities-a-voice-in-resilience

Kumar, A., & Motwani, J. (1995). A methodology for assessing time-based competitive advantage of manufacturing firms. International Journal of Operations & Production Management, 15(2), 36-53.

Mathiyalakan, S., Ashrafi, N., Zhang, W., Waage, F., Kuilboer, J.-P., & Heimann, D. (2005). Defining business agility: an exploratory study. In Proceedings of the 16th Information Resources Management Conference, San Diego, pp. 15–18.

Menor, L.J., Roth, A.V., & Mason, C.H. (2001). Agility in retail banking: A numerical taxonomy of strategic service groups. Manufacturing & Service Operations Management, 3, 273-292.

Mitchell, T. & Harris, K. (2012). Resilience: a risk management approach. Overseas,Development & Institute (Eds), ODI Background Note, Overseas Development Institute, London, p. 7.

Mitchell, T. & Harris, K. (2012). Resilience: A risk management approach. ODI Background Notes, London. Available online: http://www.odi.org.uk/sites/ odi.org.uk/files/odi-assets/publications-opinionfiles/7552.pdf

Moberg, F. & Simonsen, S.H. (2011). What is resilience? An introduction to social-ecological research. Stockholm Resilience Centre.

Montalbano, P. (2011). Trade openness and developing countries' vulnerability: Concepts, misconceptions, and directions for research. World Development, 39, 1489-1502.

Otobi, O.G. (2010). Untapped potential: how the sphere minimum standards for disaster response could promote human and institutional resilience in Northern Uganda. Resilience: Interdisciplinary Perspectives on Science and Humanitarianism, 1, pp. 61-76.

Oxfam. (2009). People-Centred Resilience: Working with Vulnerable Farmers towards Climate Change Adaptation and Food Security. Oxford, UK: Oxfam International.

Pain, A., & Levine, S. (2012). A Conceptual Analysis of Livelihoods and Resilience: Addressing the "Insecurity of Agency". HPG Work Paper, p.18.

Pregenzer A. (2011). Systems resilience: A new analytical framework for nuclear nonproliferation, Albuquerque, NM: Sandia National Laboratories.

Ramasesh, R., Kulkarni, S., & Jayakumar, M. (2001). Agility in manufacturing systems: an exploratory modeling framework and simulation. Integrated Manufacturing Systems, 12(7), pp.534-548.

Raschke, R.L., & David, J.S. (2005). Business process agility. Omaha, Ne: Eleventh Americas Conference on Information Systems.

Ross, J. W. (2008). Innovation vs. agility: the path to profitable growth: MIT Sloan CISR.

Sambamurthy, V., Bharadwaj, A., & Grover, V. (2003). Shaping Agility through Digital Options: Reconceptualizing the Role of Information Technology in Contemporary Firms. MIS Quarterly, 27(2), 237-263.

Verikios, G., Sullivan, M., Stojanovski, P., Giesecke, J., & Woo, G. (2015). Assessing Regional Risks from Pandemic Influenza: A Scenario Analysis. The World Economy.

Vugrin E.D, Warren D.E, Ehlen M.A, & Camphouse R.C. (2010). A framework for assessing the resilience of infrastructure and economic systems. Sustainable Infrastructure Systems: simulation, modeling, and intelligent engineering (pp. 77-116). Berlin: Springer-Verlag, Inc.

Walker, B.H, Holling, C.S., Carpenter, S.R., & Kinzig, A. (2004). Resilience, adaptability, and transformability in social-ecological systems. Ecology and Society, 9(2), pp. 5.

Wenzel, M, Stanske, S, & Lieberman, M.B. (2020). Strategic responses to crisis. Strategic Management Journal, 41, 7-18.

Yusuf, Y.Y., Sarhadi, M., Gunasekaran, A. (1999). Agile manufacturing: The drivers, concepts, and attributes. International Journal of Production Economics, 62, pp. 33-43.

Zhang, Z. & Sharif, H. (2000). A methodology for achieving agility in manufacturing organisations. International Journal of Operations & Production Management, 20(4), pp. 496-512.

CHAPTER 2

COVID-19: A Fast-Tracked Call for Manufacturing Industry 4.0?

Kesavan Nallaluthan & V.Sethuprakhash

2.1 Introduction

2.2 Malaysia Manufacturing Industry

2.3 Impact Of Covid-19 Pandemic on the Manufacturing Industry

    2.3.1 Background Information on COVID-19

    2.3.2 Impact of COVID-19 Pandemic on the Malaysian Manufacturing Sector

2.4 Role of Industrial 4.0

    2.4.1 Industrial Revolution (IR 4.0) and Its Elements

    2.4.2 Malaysia Board of Technologists (MBOT) and Industry

    2.4.3 Engagement

    2.4.4 Industry 4.0 Technologies and Their Applications in Fighting COVID-19

2.5 Current Strategies and Action Taken by Government to Help Manufacturing Sectors

2.6 Conclusion

2.1 INTRODUCTION

Manufacturing is a process of creating products using hands or a computer by a company which then will be sold to a consumer. Raw materials or parts of a larger product can be used in manufacturing. Manufacturing is usually carried out on a large-scale production line using sophisticated equipment and skilled labor. However, the fourth wave of industry calls for an industrial revolution that integrates automation and robotics into the seams of a manufacturing base. It is critical to reduce human error which will allow all the companies to refocus on their efforts to generate revenue. It promotes and encourages continuous improvement in manufacturing processes and establishes local market standards for achieving high-quality production, and productive practices, and increases profit opportunities for companies. However, most of the manufacturing firms are still pending implementations of Industry 4.0 due to a lack of knowledge handling it and some concern about the cybersecurity process when involving storage data in cloud systems.

Therefore the challenges faced by the manufacturing sectors have a big impact on the labor force due to movement control, supply chain disruptions, productivity, and many more due to the COVID-19 pandemic. Due to these circumstances, is this a sign of a fast-track call or activation for industry 4.0 technologies?

This chapter is organized by firstly presenting the Malaysian manufacturing industry and followed by the Impact of the Covid-19 Pandemic on the Manufacturing Industry. The third section explains the role of industry 4.0. The next section discusses the Current Strategies and Action Taken by Government to Help Manufacturing Sectors and the final section of this chapter provides the conclusion/s drawn from the study.

2.2 MALAYSIA MANUFACTURING INDUSTRY

The manufacturing industry has been the backbone of the Malaysian economy for many years. Looking back at history, rubber plantations and tin mining were the pioneers. As Malaysians, we know that our country is blessed with an abundance of natural resources with an advantage of population profile, principally workforce's age, and education levels. There are a variety of commodities such as palm oil, petroleum, rubber, and tin. At present, these commodities have evolved into manufacturing. The manufacturing sector in Malaysia can be divided into a few parts which are electrical, electronic, chemicals, machinery, and equipment. Data from all over the world shows that the manufacturing industry is growing rapidly over the years. This growth is also visible in Malaysia and the evidence of it is their manufacturing industry which has been the main sector economically for many years.

The manufacturing industry has played a vital role in the economic transformation in Malaysia. Industries such as rubber, palm oil, and tin which can be seen in the manufacturing industry in Malaysia are some of the successful industries in recent years. Other than that, manufacturing in Malaysia also includes petroleum, chemical, food, beverages, tobacco, electrical and electronic industries. According to the Department of Statistics Malaysia (2018), the manufacturing landscape in Malaysia has a total of 49,101 companies, whereby 97.14% are Small and Medium Enterprises (SMEs) and 2.86% are Large establishments. Of the SME percentage, 46% are micro, 48% are small and 6% are medium enterprises with a growth rate of 6.8% in 2017 and a 21.5% share of SMEs' Gross Domestic Product (GDP).

In the present scenario even though SMEs firms dominate the manufacturing sector, the contributions by firm size here are relatively small when compare with larger manufacturing to the growth of the country's economy. Among many manufacturing businesses in Malaysia, the rubber and palm-oil business is a long-lasting industry which had been operating until now together with some other industries such as pharmacy, medical technology, electronics, and many more others. As generally known, the Malaysian currency Ringgit Malaysia (RM) is smaller when compared to the US dollar (USD), but this fact didn't stop Malaysia from having a successful car manufacturing industry which is progressing well to compete with the best factories and quality machines industries in the world to produce a highly rated car in Malaysia. In the global vision, Malaysia already has a good competitive attitude toward the manufacturing industry and the technology which is being used currently. Therefore, they feel that every Malaysian has a strong advantage to move forward in the manufacturing industry.

2.3 IMPACT OF COVID-19 PANDEMIC ON THE MANUFACTURING INDUSTRY

2.3.1 Background Information on COVID-19

The COVID-19 pandemic in Malaysia is part of the ongoing global pandemic of coronavirus disease in 2019 (COVID-19), which is caused by a coronavirus that causes extreme acute respiratory syndrome (SARS-CoV-2). Director-General of Health Noor Hisham Abdullah oversaw the medical response and preparedness to fight the disease outbreak in Malaysia, which happened under two administrations: one of the Ministry of Health (undertaken by his immediate predecessors) and another during his tenure in office. The first cases of the SARS virus in Malaysia occurred on 25 January among Chinese tourists who had traveled to Johor from Singapore. When the epidemic initially only affected people who had recently arrived from other countries, several distinct local outbreaks arose in March of the disease during that year. A well-known example of intervention was the massive surge in Malay religious Tablighi Jamaat groups in Kuala Lumpur, and the overflow in cases in neighboring countries. By the end of March, the end of the month, over 2,000 active cases in every state and territory in the country had been added to the list of confirmed cases.

As a result of the increasing number of cases, the Malaysian Prime Minister implemented nationwide Movement Control and went into lockdown on March 18. This movement control was known as "Order" (of nationwide Movement Control) which was announced by Tan Sri Muhyiddin Yassin and together with that, the new law enforcement operations launched on March 18, which resulted in numerous new investigations done immediately. There was a slow-progressing trend in the first three months of 2020 in the number of movement control orders (MCO), but by early May 2020, there had been a decline in COVID-19 infected cases. This resulted in the removal of the "Conditional Movement" and Recovery Order phases on the same day. Although Malaysia had originally planned to end the RMCO program at the end of August, due to the detection of new cases, it was extended until the end of the year.

The third wave of COVID-19 infections occurred as a result of the Sabah state election in September 2020, several other outbreaks at Top Glove facilities throughout the rest of the year added to the situation where the number of cases increased tremendously. In response to the increased incidences of covid-19 cases from December of 2020 until the first half of 2021, the Malaysian government re-imposed CMCO and RMCO regulations across the board. Between January 2021 and February 18, the nation's healthcare system became a shell of itself, with numerous restrictions had been placed during MCOs. After that, they were only used in some states and federal territories and for several more periods, from February 18 and continuing until March 2021. As Yang di-Pertuan Agong declared a state of emergency, the Parliament and state legislatures were also ordered to remain in session for the entire year ahead of schedule, from 12th of January 2021 to 1st of August 2021, and His Highness also requested that the COVID-19 grant him additional powers until the state of Malaysia ended.

According to the findings, by March, the number of new cases had already decreased dramatically and these data made the government relax its mass-communication regulations in most states and territories. In addition to that immunizing all of its citizens was the main priority and Malaysia also started a non-citizen people COVID-19 vaccination approach in February. Thanks to that program non-residents also achieved the same level of protection from the virus on February 21, 2021. After that in the middle of April, multiple states began reporting an increase in the number of cases per day, states under MCO restrictions had also shown an increase in number. Due to the rising levels of the new cases of the highly contagious SARS-CoV-2 variants found in Malaysia, the federal government reintroduced the more widespread MCO (an emergency situation-expanding biological public health measure) between May 12th and June 7th, 2021, as per the previous plans.

In Malaysia total of 461,500 confirmed cases, which ranks fourth in the number of deaths and nearly 42,000 cases, and Indonesia comes in second, ahead in the overall number of Indonesia; Myanmar is the leading instance in Southeast Asia in total cases.

2.3.2 Impact of COVID-19 Pandemic on the Malaysian Manufacturing Sector

This pandemic not only poses a great threat to human life but also caused the economy to face a tough moment. In some countries, their government ordered a national lockdown. Meanwhile, in Malaysia, it is called the Movement Control Order, which restricts everyone from going out without a good reason. With this restriction, many businesses, factories, and manufacturers need to shut their operations during the MCO period to help to stop the spread of this disease. Many sectors were affected severely especially tourism and manufacturing as not all manufacturers are essential. The Malaysian manufacturing sector like other sectors is also affected by the COVID-19 pandemic.

Although the Malaysian Government introduces a stimulus package of USD 4.8 billion during the outbreak of COVID-19, it still was not enough to cover the loss that occurred to many people or many sectors. The pandemic has brought many changes to the manufacturing sector in our country. The most obvious impact would be the financial drawback faced by the manufacturing sector due to the COVID-19 pandemic. This sudden change in the world caused economic and financial "damage", demand cut-back, disruption of the supply chain, and troubling employment statuses in Malaysia's manufacturing sector.

The current scenario is very crucial for Malaysia because the World Bank Malaysia Economic Monitor stated that Malaysia's economy is forecasted to contract by 3.1 percent in 2020. This is due to the very sharp slowdown in economic activities due to the pandemic. The slowdown in economic activities which is partially due to weak external demands caused Malaysia's export of goods and services to be reduced for a third consecutive quarter by 7.1 percent in Q1 2020. This would be the largest decline so far since 2009's Global Financial Crisis. The slowing down of external demands for goods and services therefore directly impacts the manufacturing sector in Malaysia negatively.

Malaysia's GDP is in a critical situation whereby in a non-pandemic situation the manufacturing sector could contribute up to RM 316 billion of GDP to the Malaysian economy which comprises 22.3 percent of the national GDP of RM 1.4 trillion. However, since the COVID-19 pandemic outbreak, the potential losses of RM 12.9 billion or more have occurred during the first 14 days of the Movement Control Order. This shows that the GDP level may decrease even more drastically if the COVID-19 situations remain unchanged which affects the manufacturing industry in Malaysia.

The COVID-19 pandemic impact can also be seen through the decreasing employment rate in many sectors, especially in the manufacturing industry. There are many manufacturing companies in Malaysia where their workers lost their jobs due to the rapid economic slowdown and fast diminishing. For example, in the automotive industry, around 600,000 people are supposedly cover both manufacturing and after-sales sectors but due to the COVID-19 pandemic, it is a grief to face the potential job losses of between 10 – 20 percent from the automotive industry. This is due to the major cut-off of production and also the decreasing sales volume from the industry.

One more industry that can be highlighted to explain further the negative impact of the COVID-19 pandemic is the logistics sector. Malaysia, which possesses one of the most important ports in the South East Asia region, is facing drawbacks in the logistics industry. This is because the reduced rate of manufactured goods and the lessened demands for the goods to be imported and exported somehow impact the logistics sector too. Due to the outburst of the pandemic, the contribution of the GDP of the logistics sector has decreased to RM 57 billion only which is 41 percent of the national GDP of RM 4.1 trillion. In addition to that, the employment amount figuratively is at 437,926 is also more likely to decrease impacting many lower-wage employees of the logistics sector such as drivers, equipment operators and clerical staff by either the company retrenching them or the company had to be closed down due to economic constraints. Although there are many negative impacts of COVID-19 on the manufacturing sector in Malaysia, the positive impacts should be taken into account too. One of the most important manufacturing sectors which boost Malaysia's economy is the glove sector. The emergence of the COVID-19 pandemic has put the glove manufacturer in the driving seat. The increase in demand for the gloves to be used by everyone during this crucial time had made the Bursa Malaysia listed glove makers be a catalyst whereby the flurry of the buying activity has pushed their share price up by 10 percent to 68 percent this year to date.

For example, the world's largest rubber glove manufacturer, Top Glove Corporation Berhad stated that the sales volume has doubled since February 2020. Moreover, according to The Malaysian Rubber Glove Manufacturers Association, the global expectation of the demand for gloves will surge by 20 percent to 25 percent in the interim. Food supply is so important during this pandemic season. Since the Malaysian government announced the Movement Control Order, people are forbidden from dining out. Knowing the circumstances of the MCO, people have begun to embark on panic buying of food supplies. The most popular food product that gets snapped away immediately is bread. The most well-known food manufacturing company, Gardenia could not cope with the high demand from customers during the ongoing MCO period. According to Gardenia Bakeries (KL) Sdn Bhd, the manufacturing or production of loaves of bread has increased to 2.2 million a day through a total of 5 factories operating 24 hours a day. These increasing demands for the manufacturing of food chain supplies somehow have contributed to the margin of the Malaysian economy.

Generally, manufacturing is the prime sector in Malaysia. A lot of foreign companies make direct investments in all kinds of industries. This has helped Malaysia to boost the Gross Domestic Product (GDP) and also, employment. However, due to this pandemic, they lose a massive amount of revenue when all operations need to be stopped during MCO. Many companies are facing financial struggles with this restriction. These companies have to bear the massive loss in revenue. Consequently, they have to retrench their employees who are surplus, or in a worst-case scenario, they have to shut down the entire operation for good. The Department of Statistics Malaysia revealed that Malaysia's GDP has declined badly (17.1%) and it is recorded as the lowest since it's shrunk from the fourth quarter of 1998 (11.2%). Besides, the manufacturing statistics also revealed the sales value during April plunged to RM 75.8 billion as compared to the previous month which was RM 110 billion.

Therefore, there is also a significant impact of COVID-19 on crude oil prices. The oil price has slumped during early March and it has bounced back from below USD 20 per barrel to somewhat above USD 30 per barrel.

2.4 ROLE OF INDUSTRIAL REVOLUTION 4.0

2.4.1 Industrial Revolution (IR 4.0) and Its Elements

The first industrial revolution began in the 18th century and now we are approaching the fourth industrial revolution, also known as (IR 4.0). Industry Revolution 4.0 is things that focus on interconnectivity, automation, machine learning, and real-time data. Sometimes, they also refer to IoT or smart manufacturing, physical production, and operations with smart digital technology, machine learning, and big data to create a more holistic and better-connected ecosystem for companies that focus on manufacturing and supply chain management. Every company and organization's operating system is will be different. They will face a different kind of challenge, so that is where Industry Revolution 4.0 will play its role. Industry Revolution 4.0 is something that invests in new technology and tools to improve manufacturing efficiency, but they will make a revolution in the way how the business operates and grows. Why it is called Industry Revolution 4.0? It is because this Industry Revolution has four phases. The First Industrial Revolution begins in the 18th century. During this period they focus more on manual labor performed by the people and work animals. The Second Industrial Revolution occurred in the 20th century when they introduced steel and the use of electricity in factories. This new introduction has made the manufacturers increase their efficiency and make the factory machine a better machine. During this time, it boosted productivity.

The Third Industry Revolution started in the 1950s through partial automation using memory-programmable controls and computers. Since this technology is introduced, many machines were able to automate the production process without human assistance. Robots are good examples that perform as programmed entities without human intervention. The fourth one is last but not least which is the Fourth Industrial Revolution going on in this current era. During this time digital technology from recent decades reached a whole new level with the help of interconnectivity through the Internet of Things (IoT), access to real-time data, and the introduction of cyber-physical systems. It connects physically with digital and allows for better collaboration and access across departments, partners, vendors, products, and people. Industry 4.0 empowers business owners to better control and understands every aspect of their operation and allows them to leverage instant data to boost productivity, improve processes, and drive growth.

Industry 4.0 is all about data integration, artificial intelligence, machinery, and communication to create a highly efficient industrial ecosystem that is not just automated but intelligent, to provide satisfying goods and services. There are nine elements of Industry 4.0. First is, Big Data which means a large volume of data that swamps a business daily. However, it is not about the amount of data, but how can it be analyzed for insights that can recognize patterns. This element is cost-efficient and good in reducing errors. Also, it is useful to make a decision when planning a strategy based on the data collected.

The second element is a simulation and this element can simulate a virtual environment of the factory itself with real-time data and analyze the productivity before a change in the factory can be made. Also, it aids in making the best decision and design visualization. With design visualization, engineers can detect early issues or obstacles from the design. The third is horizontal and vertical integration. Horizontal integration takes networking among the cyber-physical systems to a whole new level. Each device and system at the same level of manufacturing is connected which makes communication between systems way easier.

In this way, the task can be managed by the machines themselves. Meanwhile, vertical integration enables everyone in the company including the system to have all the data with the required abstraction. Internet of Things (IoT) is the next element that is a very important element for the manufacturing industry. It is an ecosystem in which all the sensors and actuators can function separately and communicate with every other element. It is useful because if an employee overlooked something, the machinery can be stopped automatically. Furthermore, autonomous robots work similarly to humans but with an additional feature which is, that they operate based on a complex logic algorithm. This means they do not need any pre-set path to do their part. Cloud is the next element that acts as a remote system that allows users to access information stored anywhere using the internet. It facilitates the businesses in their operations. The information is safely stored with backup and easily accessed whenever there is an internet connection. It also provides real-time data and allows people with credentials to have access to this cloud.

Cybersecurity is another element that gives confidence to people in this 4th industrial evolution. Increased connectivity in the system poses a threat to a particular company. Cybersecurity acts as protection from theft or hackers. Lastly, additive manufacturing like 3D printing is used to make prototypes and proof of concepts. This technological advancement allows us to design complex designs which seem impossible to do with conventional manufacturing processes.

2.4.2 Malaysia Board of Technologists (MBOT) and Industry 4.0 Engagement

The MBOT was incorporated in November 2016 as a technical organization dedicated to recognizing technologists and technicians as professionals. This comes into effect after the Malaysian Parliament gazetted the Technologists and Technicians Act 2015 (Act 768) 2015. It should be remembered that as Malaysia prepares for industry 4.0, it is critical to recognize the positions and obligations of technologists and technicians.

MBOT strives to be among the world's leading nations in terms of domestic economic growth, and technological progress. Industry 4.0 places a premium on innovations. Industry 4.0 incorporates forward-thinking concepts such as the Internet of Things (IoT), 3D printing, autonomous vehicles, biotechnology, and nanotechnology. Jobs in Malaysia have shifted due to emerging technologies. Sufficient professional human capital to run emerging technology is critical for a country like Malaysia to continue developing. Several new career styles include mastery of novel tasks. However, it must be stated that innovations do not eliminate the need for technologists.

Rather than that, they inspire them to perform their duties. Technologists make use of human abilities and traits such as intellect, imagination, and knowledge that robots cannot reproduce. This is the mindset of MBOT for all to embrace.

As a result, MBOT accelerates its progress to provide graduates with the skills necessary to meet the country's aspirations. If MBOT can not address issues appropriately and effectively, they will not be where they want to be in the future. Therefore, they should be adequately armed.

MBOT is critical in advancing the government's National Science, Technology, Engineering, and Maths (STEM) agenda as in the Malaysia Education Blueprint 2013 – 2025. As is, the percentage of secondary students studying STEM subjects hovers around 27%. However, as Technical and Vocational Education and Training (TVET) is used, the percentage increases to 47%, which is promising. The nation needs more high-quality STEM graduates to propel the country forward. Numerous aspects must be addressed for MBOT to soar to new heights amid Industry 4.0. MBOT looks forward to everyone's assistance and helps in further developing MBOT and carrying out what has been charted. MBOT values everyone's continued contribution in assisting MBOT in producing a significant impact on the nation as a whole in Industry 4.0 engagement.

2.4.3 Industry 4.0 Technologies and Their Applications in Fighting COVID-19

Industry 4.0 emphasizes the significance of data collection and sharing in the value chain by incorporating increasingly intelligent, autonomous, and automated production systems. Industry 4.0 is a term that refers to the fusion of information and communication technologies (ICT) and industrial technology. Numerous businesses are implementing innovations such as Cyber-Physical Systems (CPS), the Internet of Things (IoT), robotics, big data, cloud manufacturing, and augmented reality to enhance products and processes, increase performance and productivity, minimize costs, and boost customer loyalty. Numerous benefits accrue to businesses as a result of Industry 4.0: increased versatility and speed from prototype to series production; increased efficiency as a result of shorter set-up times, decreased defects, and system downtime; and improved quality and waste reduction. Additionally, incidents can be avoided in the workplace by incorporating Industry 4.0 technology into safety management systems.

Since the outbreak of the pandemic, manufacturers have been debating how Industry 4.0 would help mitigate the crisis's impact. To begin, Industry 4.0 has the potential to alter the way we function. The trend toward remote work will accelerate and could be aided by Industry 4.0. However, remote working is not synonymous with working from home; it entails a fundamental restructuring of the organizational structure. The most drastic effect of Industry 4.0 is the dematerialization of the workplace, which ensures that some tasks can be conducted using digital equipment linked to the Internet, allowing employees to perform their duties in locations other than company buildings. Before the pandemic, working from home was considered appropriate only in the information technology and technology fields. Over the past few months, businesses from a variety of industries have discovered the advantages of remote work and are considering it as a new business model due to the impact of the COVID-19 pandemic

Remote working is not a new phenomenon. It has started way before the lockdown scenario arose and it has gained popularity in developed countries. The primary benefits are including time savings, increased satisfaction with work organization, and the improvement of leadership and teamwork skills. These facts were supported by the case in Italy as reported by Lepore et al. (2021). In his article, the Italian General Confederation of Labour's (CGIL) and Di Vittorio Foundation's "smart working" survey incorporates this data, estimating that approximately 500,000 people worked remotely before the epidemic. Before the COVID-19 lockout, remote jobs in Italy were a small percentage of the workforce, accounting for just 1.2 percent of total employment. The percentage increased to 8.8 after the quarantine, with peaks of 50% in sectors such as communication and information and 40% in technological and research activities.

However, the option varied by firm size and sector: remote working was used in 18.3 percent of cases in the smallest companies, but up to 90 percent in the largest. In recent months, the Politecnico di Milano's Smart working Observatory reported that 8 million Italians work remotely. Remote work is also expected to contribute to sustainable growth, as shown by the potential contribution of remote work in addressing energy and environmental challenges. In this situation, digital technology that enables remote work will help more companies thrive and resume normal operations. Numerous studies have examined the effect of Industry 4.0 technology on manufacturing, the labor market, and culture during the pandemic, showing how the virus accelerated advancements in emerging technologies. Additionally, as Industry 4.0 developments accelerate, significant opportunities for sustainable manufacturing will emerge.

According to some researchers, Big Data would drive sustainable development in the future of Industry 4.0 applications, especially concerning the United Nations (UN) Sustainable Development Goals (SDGs) adopted in 2015. Braccini and Margherita demonstrate through a case study of a manufacturing business that Industry 4.0 applications can promote economic, social, and environmental sustainability. Precisely, by allowing virtualization, digitization, and automation, Industry 4.0 will increase environmental awareness, thereby reducing waste and maximizing the use of natural resources, raw materials, and energy. Despite the advantages of Industry 4.0 for smart and sustainable production, the majority of businesses have made no progress toward implementation.

Table 2.1 summarises the applications of Industry 4.0 in the post-COVID-19 recovery phase, based on the most recent literature on the relationship between Industry 4.0 and COVID-19. Table 2.1 illustrates how Industry 4.0 can incorporate COVID-19 effects by leveraging data, computing power, and connectivity. Rapid change necessitates rethinking existing business models, which is vital for enhancing "digital resilience," a critical factor in firms' performance. SMEs may consider sharing the costs associated with technology investments across collaborative networks to gain access to innovation and broader knowledge bases. Industry 4.0 trends have the potential to accelerate the adoption of sustainable business models in SMEs, thereby improving their efficiency.

Table 2.1 Applications of Industry 4.0 in the post-COVID-19 recovery phase

4.0 Enabling Technologies	Potential Applications in Industry
Advanced Manufacturing Solutions	• Robots can be deployed and equipped to perform routine activities, effectively socially distancing themselves from humans. • Sensors worn by employees will track COVID-19 symptoms in real-time. • Chatbots are capable of responding to a wide variety of questions from the general public and customers.
Additive Manufacturing	• 3D printing enables the production of high-demand goods and essential components that are currently unavailable from suppliers. The technology has the potential to contain the virus's spread through the manufacture of face masks. • 3D scanning can be used in a variety of applications, including motion capture, robotic mapping, and industrial design.
Augmented Reality	• Virtual and augmented reality technologies bridge the physical divide between individuals, enabling them to collaborate and provide instructions in a nearly "real-life" environment.

4.0 Enabling Technologies	Potential Applications in Industry
Simulation	• Artificial intelligence-enabled systems will assist businesses in simulating live-work environments and establishing on-demand labor forces. • Virtual Reality (VR) enhances teamwork performance, eliminates travel costs, and mitigates the environmental effects of emissions. Virtual reality is a means of contact and collaboration.
Horizontal/ Vertical Integration	• Intelligent information management systems powered by artificial intelligence combine and disseminate knowledge across the supply chain, thus motivating employees.
Industrial Internet and Cloud	• Cloud-based management software enables businesses to remotely track and manage processes and equipment. • IoT may be used in conjunction with drones to conduct surveillance, trace the source of an outbreak, or locate patient zero. Then, medical personnel may use IoT to track patients remotely at home.
Cyber-security	• When asset downtime is large or activities are shut down, businesses should enhance cybersecurity at all levels.

4.0 Enabling Technologies	Potential Applications in Industry
Big Data and Analytics	• Internet of Things-based software creates a real-time dashboard of key performance metrics to facilitate shop-floor performance dialogues and improve transparency. The data collected could provide details about the current and historical state of the machine, as well as customer records. • Big data can be beneficial for predicting the virus's effect on business, gathering real-time data, and delivering this data to managers to help them plan a response strategy.

Source: Lepore et al. (2021)

2.5 CURRENT STRATEGIES AND ACTION TAKEN BY THE GOVERNMENT TO HELP MANUFACTURING SECTORS

Under the circumstance of a global pandemic that crippled not only the human body but also global politics and the economy. The Malaysian economy is also not exempted from catastrophic events. However, due to the government which was quick in making impromptu decisions, they were able to sustain themselves in rebalancing the economy despite receiving limited help from first-world countries such as the USA, China, and Australia. This saved local manufacturers from going out of business. In the manufacturing sector, there are mostly local companies that were affected by COVID-19 which caused all operations to come to a crawl, if not a halt. Thus, after receiving an early warning of the pandemic sweep, the government was appealed to on issuing a bill to save the small retailers and manufacturers. The government then enacted a new COVID-19 bill comparable to that of Singapore and the UK. The bill was issued to provide aid to the manufacturers for them to endure the staggering economy so that they would be able to move on with their operations post-pandemic.

The second strategy implied by the government was the second stimulus package for SMEs as well as manufacturers. The stimulus package worth RM 250 billion was given out as fiscal injections towards manufacturers so that they have some equity so which will help them from running out of funds and resources to keep their businesses up and operating.

Due to COVID-19, people tend to save money more than spend it, thus, avoiding buying for most "wants", and some do not even spend money on their "needs". With financial aid from the government via the stimulus package, these manufacturers can maintain operations despite not having sales, pre-Covid?. The third strategy is that government officials decided to help care for society's mental health by urging manufacturers, business owners, and employees to calm down and settle things together rather than having the manufacturers fail their employees by not paying them, forcing leaves, salary cuts and retrench them without a solid reason. Based on Myanmar's labors, they discussed between themselves the pandemic and the problems they are facing until they reach a unanimous decision. Such fluid communication is vital for the whole manufacturing hierarchy to flourish and might even be able to perform better regardless of whatever situation. Another strategy implemented by the government is to also provide special loans for manufacturers to borrow. Such loans come in with much lower interest rates and smaller payment amounts which benefit manufacturers as a whole.

This strategy allows businesses that produce and manufacture goods daily to relax a bit on their transactional and financial issues, thus, improving performance, increasing sales, and the relaxation of workers. This is meant to assure workers will not face any negative scenario all of a sudden despite their hard work given to the manufacturer. As mentioned before, employees within Malaysia are facing negative feedback towards their work currently, whereby they are on the brink of losing their jobs, or maybe their wages. Due to this, the government found a solution by strengthening the labor laws. The enforcement of upgrading the labor laws could protect the employees at the very least. It is understood that the economy is declining, but this is considered an inevitable event and manufacturers do not have the right to chuck off or mistreat their employees under the excuse that they are facing an economic downfall. By strengthening labor laws, it could be assured that the government has one less problem to deal with, which is the protection of the employees in the manufacturing sector. The final strategy used by the government in helping manufacturers is by regulating the policies and rates issued by the Central Bank, or Bank Negara Malaysia. By lowering the policy rates not only for personal borrowers but also for small, medium, and corporations, borrowers obtained the luxury of flexibility where they do not have to rake up money to only pay loans with whatever money they have and earn during these dire times.

For example, the pharmaceutical sector, which is also a manufacturing sector where drugs and medicine are made in Malaysia under the close monitoring of the Medicinal Board and the Health Ministry, can divert their funding into production costs, and employee earnings as well as research funding. In terms of finance, when a company that is listed and has shared their company worth, with the lax loan payments and lower policy rates, such companies can tap into their equity funding into investing in better products, or even a vaccine in regards to the pandemic we are facing right now. This strategy is simply saying more money, fewer payments, fewer costs, and better manufacturing. In conclusion, the government has provided a vast amount of subsidies and aid to keep manufacturing businesses running and performing well despite being washed by the global economic downturn. Such strategies are more than beneficial for manufacturers to produce goods like normal.

2.6 CONCLUSION

This chapter presents activation for Industry 4.0 in the manufacturing sector as a fast track due to the current COVID-19 pandemic. If there is no manufacturing it will be difficult for humans to produce goods. Manufacturing is a process to produce things for humans to provide for the basic needs of their lives. Most of the raw materials are converted to usable products after going through manufacturing. Almost all sectors in our country produce goods through manufacturers.

The manufacturing sector generates a huge amount of revenue for our country each year. Manufacturers from other countries have built many manufacturing companies in Malaysia such as electronic companies or automotive companies. For instance, electronic products are largely exported from our country. The usage of Industry 4.0 in the manufacturing industry increases the competitiveness of the manufacturing industry. The technology of Industry 4.0 helps manufacturers to produce goods efficiently. For example, all the data can be stored systematically and accordingly with the use of technology from Industry 4.0. The production of goods can be done without the use of the huge hard work of the employee. Industry 4.0 has significantly affected the production ways of goods in many ways in the production industry.

In the manufacturing sector, Industry 4.0 technology has deliberately been used since Industry 4.0 began. Many people in our country have been trained to utilize Industry 4.0 technology well. People have graduated or trained in the various fields that contribute to the usage of technologies in Industry 4.0. For example, to operate the systems people will be trained. Talented people can bring the usage of Industry 4.0 technology to the next level in the manufacturing industry. Industry 4.0 technology has been very useful to the manufacturing processes in various ways. It has contributed largely to the manufacturing industry in Malaysia. In the developmental process of our country technology has played its role also. Incorporating technology Industry 4.0 in the manufacturing sector has helped manufacturers in dealing with problems and becoming more flexible.

Many manufacturers in Malaysia are aware of Industry 4.0 and it is a fast track for combating the COVID-19 pandemic. However, not many of them are ready to adopt this modern technology as listed in Table 1. There are multiple reasons behind this not readiness. One of them would be the lack of a skilled workforce. To adopt this concept, companies need to ensure that their employees have the necessary skill to work with the machinery. Training programs should be provided by the human resource department. Apart from that, managers also need to equip themselves with Industry 4.0 knowledge by attending any seminar regarding it and transferring the knowledge to the employees. This will keep the employees to be well aware of current technology, especially in increasing productivity at work.

Industry 4.0 can bring a significant impact on the Malaysian manufacturing industry. When a local manufacturer starts going digital and fully adopts Industry 4.0, the quality of the products can be improved tremendously. In return, the consumer will be more satisfied and gain more trust in local goods. Also, it can help in reducing error rates with the data from the sensor which can minimize loss. Nevertheless, Industry 4.0 can also bring a negative impact because when manufacturers depend fully on technologies, some employees are not needed anymore. After all, the machinery has replaced them. All in all, can conclude that moving towards the fourth industrial revolution brings more benefits than harm. Meanwhile, many scholars from various disciplines welcomed to research Industry 4.0 technologies to support local manufacturers to make them more confident when engaged in. Therefore, this is the right time as the fast track to activation of Industry 4.0 in the manufacturing sectors.

ACKNOWLEDGEMENT

We would like to thank everyone who contributed directly or indirectly to the chapter contents.

REFERENCES

COVID-19 pandemic in Malaysia - Wikipedia. (n.d.). Retrieved May 16, 2021, from https://en.wikipedia.org/wiki/COVID-19_pandemic_in_Malaysia

Deloitte. Smart Operations in Time of COVID-19 Innovative Ways to Keep the Business Running 2020. Available online https://www2.deloitte.com/nl/nl/pages/energy_resources industrials/articles/industry40-smart-operations in-time-of-COVID-19.html (accessed on 15 May 2020).

Czifra, G., & Molnár, Z. (2020). Covid-19 and Industry 4.0. Research Papers Faculty of Materials Science and Technology Slovak *University of Technology, 28*(46), 36–45. https://doi.org/10.2478/rput-2020-0005

Javaid, M., Haleem, A., Vaishya, R., Bahl, S., Suman, R., & Vaish, A. (2020). Industry 4.0 technologies and their applications in fighting COVID-19 pandemic. *Diabetes & Metabolic Syndrome: Clinical Research & Reviews, 14*(4), 419–422. https://doi.org/10.1016/j.dsx.2020.04.032

Lepore, D., Micozzi, A., & Spigarelli, F. (2021). Industry 4.0 Accelerating Sustainable Manufacturing in the COVID-19 Era: Assessing the Readiness and Responsiveness of Italian Regions. *Sustainability, 13*(5), 2670. https://doi.org/10.3390/su13052670

Mckinsey & Company. Coronavirus: Industrial IoT in Challenging Times 2020. Available online: https://www.mckinsey.com/ industries/advanced electronics/our-insights/coronavirus-industrial-IoT-in challenging-times (accessed on 15 May 2021).

Mohamad, E., Sukarma, L., Mohamad, N. A., Salleh, M. R., Rahman, M. A. A., Rahman, A. A. A., & Sulaiman, M. A. (2018). Review on Implementation of Industry 4.0 Globally and Preparing Malaysia for Fourth Industrial Revolution. *The Proceedings of Design & Systems Conference, 2018.28*(0), 2203. https://doi.org/10.1299/jsmedsd.2018.28.2203

Oztemel, E., & Gursev, S. (2020). Literature review of Industry 4.0 and related technologies. *Journal of Intelligent Manufacturing, 31*(1), 127–182. https://doi.org/10.1007/s10845-018-1433-8

President's Notes of Malaysia Board of Technologists (MBOT), Techies, Official Bulletin 4th Edition

Sarkis, J., Cohen, M. J., Dewick, P., & Schröder, P. (2020b). A brave new world: Lessons from the COVID-19 pandemic for transitioning to sustainable supply and production. *Resources, Conservation and Recycling,* 159, 104894. https://doi.org/10.1016/j.resconrec.2020.104894

Sipalan, J., & Holmes, S. (2020). Malaysia confirms first cases of coronavirus infection. *Reuters.* https://www.reuters.com/article/china-health-malaysia/malaysia-confirms-first-cases-of-coronavirus-infection-idUSL4N29U03A

CHAPTER 3

Airlines: The Broken Wings

Uma Shangery Aruldass

3.1 INTRODUCTION

In this chapter, the author begins by discussing the reality of COVID-19 in the airline industry and its impact. The author has also highlighted the actions needed to restore the industry from the pandemic and followed by the future actions needed to create a sustainable airline industry. The author has shared her personal experience of surviving the pandemic and other pandemic-related crises. The airline industry will overcome the hit with clear plans and negotiations with the stakeholders.

3.2 COVID-19 IN THE AIRLINE INDUSTRY

The metal birds are resting on the tarmac. The runaway is strikingly less congested for an international airport. The skies are empty. The aircrafts had nowhere to go. The sound of the wind breeze was audible! These are extremely hard times for the airline industry. COVID-19 has had a devastating effect on the airline industry. This statement had been covered by numerous newspapers from all over the world as their headlines. Between March and April 2020, every word, sentence, and front-page covers COVID-19. The airline industry is defined as a business that transports passengers who pay for the service and freight via air space through systematically scheduled routes, mainly by airplanes and also by helicopters. The airline industry is an expensive industry to live in. The liabilities are extremely high and beyond imagination for many. The skillsets needed to serve the airline industry are niche and the job markets are in 'highly-paid' categories. Travelling by airplane has become more affordable in recent years, particularly with the rise of low-cost airlines. According to International Civil Aviation Organization (ICAO), the number of world passenger traffic (international and domestic travelers) from 2009 to 2019 has increased to 2,150 million passengers, or 86% growth in traffic.

All of this growth directly benefits communication between countries and physical presence in those countries.

3.3 COVID-19'S EFFECT ON THE AIRLINE INDUSTRY

When it comes to airlines, the industry has taken a significant and costly hit as a result of the pandemic. The impact on the airline industry is severe and long-lasting. Airlines are barely able to breathe out of the COVID-19. Government intervention is essential to contain the spread of the disease. However, travel restrictions and border closures by the government pulled down the entire industry. Over the course of the two acts, a significant decrease in passenger demand was observed; consequently, the aircraft were grounded as well, as there were no passengers and the borders were closed. Airlines do come up with ways to scale back existing operations to remain competitive. These will be thoroughly discussed in the subsequent sub-topics.

3.3.1 Government Enforcement

To curb the spread of COVID-19, the government of each country has to come up with heavy measures like a lockdown. The COVID-19 cases are very similar to snowball effects as it increases the number of infected cases in a very short time. The disease also spreads extensively across the globe within months and it is fatal. Fatalities have been recorded up to 1 million within a year of the emergence of COVID-19.

3.3.2 Travel Restrictions

The travel restrictions have been imposed by the government of responding countries. The 14-day mandatory quarantine has been practiced by many countries as an infected individual, would develop symptoms as early as 14 days. Therefore, to stop the spread individually, the government has to introduce the mandatory quarantine with the COVID-19 test. However, there are individuals with symptomatic (individuals who develop symptoms over affected disease) and asymptomatic (individuals who do not develop symptoms of affected disease).

Due to the medical glitch in the early symptoms, governments have to proceed further with travel restrictions within the country. Most governments have also requested travel declarations from citizens departing from, entering, and travelling within the country. All of these steps have increased the cost of travel and instilled psychological fear in passengers.

Passenger Demand

Once COVID-19 has started to take a toll on the airline industry, the psychological fear among the passengers has reached its peak. Passengers were afraid of COVID-19 which lacks a vaccine. As a result, fear of the invisible virus has kept people from flying. Airline demand has also fallen precipitously, owing to the government-imposed travel restrictions. A drop in airline demand, impacts, and the number of flights scheduled simply mean losing the whole revenue stream.

Revenue Management

The revenue stream for airlines has been highly affected by the COVID-19 pandemic. Airlines have unique revenue management as airlines can stimulate the supply and demand based on revenue management strategies. However, it is harder to stimulate demand compared to supply.

The algorithms work in numerous ways at once. The data collected, and the previous data are the airline's biggest assets. The revenue will be generated based on the historical data for an airline. There are a lot of factors that control the algorithms such as days, months, festivals, seasons, and most importantly public holidays. The seat pricing is fixed based on the demand for the respective flights and routes. Additionally, pricing typically increases as the departure dates approach. If we realized that flight pricing varies throughout the day, the morning flight would cost nearly twice as much as the last flight of the day to the same destination on the same day. That does sound like a lot, doesn't it? Yes! That is how complicated a revenue management system and algorithm for an airline is because, in reality, all of the controlling factors work as one to determine a seat price.

These are the secrets for an airline on how the algorithm works. This could be done manually too especially when the demand is uncertain and when the patterns are disrupted.

Airlines do more than merely transporting people and goods from point A to point B. Airlines are also a business that has a very low-profit margin in a tough competitive industry. This is where the airlines differentiate themselves in the different business models as the premium carrier, hybrid service carrier, and low-cost carrier. The differentiation helps the airlines to clearly identify their market segments and operate accordingly. The pricing is also highly influenced by the business model of an airline.

Elasticity

Airlines are always have been elastic demand market. The algorithms used to be adjusted in a way whereby when there is a high demand, the supply will be increased. The frequencies of flights will be increased. If we've ever noticed, flight frequencies on public holidays are higher for vacation destinations such as beaches during the summer. On the other hand, during meetings, incentives, conferences, and exhibitions (MICE) are more frequencies of flights from all industrial states to the MICE venue. Simply by increasing the frequencies, the airlines will be able to increase the supply.

Disrupted Algorithms

However, during the covid-19 pandemic, the revenue management algorithms are more towards disrupted patterns. The computers that control the algorithm often get confused. This is due to the data that airlines have been referring to and the pandemic situation is no longer the same. Airlines markets are no longer elastic, it has become inelastic. The target market has become very much less sensitive to changes in pricing.

Low airfare is no longer lucrative for people to travel. Business travellers have been shifted from physical meetings to virtual meetings. Air travel has been considered unsafe by many as airports are in highly populated areas. This is an alarming situation because airlines do make money from a large number of passengers and large frequencies which results in a large number of revenues.

The pandemic has instilled fear in everyone. People have less awareness of the covid-19, too many sources of information but nothing solves the problem. Everyone merely avoids the virus by isolating it. This is when social distancing in crowded areas is the best solution at the moment. Avoiding populated areas seems to be a better resolution compared to social distance as the covid-19 has risks due to physical transmission

3.3.3 Border Closure

The crisis for airlines deepened as countries closed their borders. COVID-19 and the airline industry are very much connected as airlines are the ones that directly transport people from one country to another. In other words, airlines are the ones that run businesses by connecting one country to another. So the countries closed their borders to protect the country and also to minimize the spread through international connections. Airports designed are made in such a way to keep the aircraft in constant motion instead of stationary. The airports are never meant to be optimized by storing many aircraft. The scenario contradicts what it has been designed for.

Aircrafts Grounded

Parking the aircraft on the ground has been a hassle as the space is not able to accommodate the number of fleets. This results in aircraft being parked at taxiways, cargo terminals, and also sharing space with other nearby airports. This is one of the biggest challenges that airlines face as the location of the parking is simply not the space meant for such facilities. Taxiways are the connection route from runways to terminals. The aircraft are being squeezed immediately next to each other to park them. Squeezing in this situation is being defined as parking precisely, which is another challenge. Aircraft have different safety rules and measures to follow according to the model and made. Parking precisely, without any indication on the tarmac, keeping in mind the aircraft surrounding it as the damages will incur as simple as the engine is started and the wind being sucked and blown to the aircraft's right behind and beside it.

Engineering Duties

Even though the flights are on the ground, not flying, the engineering duties and responsibilities need to be done accordingly. Grounding aircraft for some substantial time is not optimal for aircraft and the impact might be reflected in the safety of the aircraft. Aircraft are simply not as easy as starting the engines now and flying immediately. No! Dozens of checks need to be done on the aircraft before it could take off in the air again.

Humidity

While the aircraft is on the ground, the surrounding temperature and humidity do play a threatening role. This is because a highly humid environment would promote the growth of fungus in aircraft cabins and other compartments. The easiest way to let the cabin less humid would be by allowing the sunlight to enter the cabin through the aircraft windows. However, the cabin materials would get spoiled if it gets exposed to the sunlight, therefore the cabin windows should be kept closed all while the aircraft is on the ground. The engineers have to be creative at this moment to keep the solution cheap, effective, and protective of the aircraft. This is when the silica gels are being used to place them in the compartments of the grounded aircraft. The silica gels need to be placed all over the aircraft and most importantly on the expensive aircraft engines. This silica gel works exactly like how we used to use it conventionally, absorbs the moisture in the air, and keeps the surface free from any fungi growth.

Animal Threats

Moving on, looking into the animals' threats. Aircraft on the grounds are exposed to animals from birds to insects. Any form of the animal is extremely dangerous to the aircraft. On the other hand, when aircraft are on the ground and parked without operations for a couple of weeks during this Covid-19 pandemic, that's when we can find bird nests in the lower wing areas. The areas are mostly shaded and secured by the wing structures, therefore, it has been a perfect spot for the birds to nest. The nests have to be removed carefully and placed elsewhere safely. Getting back to the aircraft, it has been a whole new experience of babysitting the birds and extra inspections on the hidden wings and fuselages need to be taken.

Engines

The engines are the most expensive parts of an aircraft. The engines are also the vulnerable parts of an aircraft when on the skies as engine failures could be fatal. The animal threats, birds might take opportunities to nest inside the engine chamber when the aircraft is grounded, therefore, the engines have to be covered perfectly with the engine covers. The engine covers come in various sizes according to the engine sizes. The engine covers are made from durable material for weather and heat. Besides animal threats, the engines are needed to be protected from the weather as well. Countries across the world differ in climates and seasons. Each aircraft need to be protected based on the currently parked geological areas.

Secured parking

The parked aircraft, need to be secured well and tight to the grounds. When the heavy wind blows, the aircraft can be moved and damages the next bay aircraft. To retain the aircraft in a safe place during windy seasons, the engineers need to add weights to the aircraft. The weights need to be added and the loadmaster will be calculating the perfect spots for the weights to be placed as the center of gravity should not be disturbed.

3.4 ACTIONS NEEDED TO TAKE OFF THE INDUSTRY

The worrisome situation will continue until medical help come in, However, waiting for a vaccine could take years. Airlines need to come up with so many new steps and creative ways to keep afloat amid the global pandemic. Again, in the competitive industry, the airlines need to react fast to not to lose the potential market and area for growth ways as follows: bailouts, economic stimulus, and growing smaller. The recovery steps are the breathers for the airlines to be back in action after a long-quarantined period.

3.4.1 Bailouts

Bailouts are extremely important for airlines to resume their services immediately. Airlines have plunged deeply into financial crisis and only capital injections from the government or individuals would keep airlines to rise. Most airlines are seeking help from government bailouts to support their pending paycheques for their employees and vendors. The government also needs to help airlines out to give tax exemptions for the services being used for idling. This is mainly on the parking fees for the aircraft. The aircraft is one of the biggest burdens as they are costly on air and ground too. The bailouts need to be used for airlines to encourage them on looking for lights in the dimmed COVID-19 situation.

The situation is in a way whereby when an aircraft needs to take off, yet it has a big amount of debts on it which makes it harder for an instant fly. Aircraft are usually always in debt, it could be either supply chain debts or leasing debts. Being in debt is not a new norm for airlines but being extensively flooded with debts is new. The debts are beyond the revenue that the aircraft would make when it flies. The cumulative amount of debts especially from the supply chain is very wide. The supply chain means the basic and luxurious necessary equipment and items for an aircraft to take off. They are inclusive of food vendors, jet fuel, cleaning services, loading and unloading, and many other crucial supports.

The individuals that would be able to help out on the bailouts could be the investors or stakeholders. The same scenario applies when the airline could use the liquid cash to survive through the debts from the pandemic. It will be hard yet airlines need to survive further with the bailouts received.

3.4.2 Economic Stimulus

The economic stimulus initiative is beneficial to swim through the drastic demand collapse within the industry. Economic stimulation is a way of keeping the airline going when there is no active revenue stream. The economic stimulus efforts can be seen in packages in terms of grants or loans to keep the daily activities going. These are such as payroll protection for the employees, bonds, and equity protection for the stakeholders to make sure the airlines do not collapse.

The other form of economic stimulus is directly dealing with the aircraft's essential supports to keep supplying the needs. This economic stimulus method varies from country to country and government to government. There are certain airlines paid more attention like flag carriers compared to the other commercial airlines in the country. This is deeply connected to the pride of the nation as well.

The initiative does include training and educational institutions in the airline industry to keep progressing and producing certified and qualified personnel. This is because, during the time of crisis, the airline industry would have had a bad image in public as it is not a sustainable industry for career growth. The industry seems very fragile and the future is very uncertain especially when another pandemic visits in near future. Therefore, the demand for training and education would have been decreased. So this issue could be solved by the economic stimulus package providing the aid to sponsor more trainees and students.

3.4.3 Grow Smaller

Most of the smaller airlines would not meet their ends at the end of the battle, the gigantic one does, by simply growing smaller. When the airline has so much on its plates, the best to do is to restructure the current management. This takes so much from the number of fleets, the number of employees, and supply chain management too.

Air travel is expensive, the longer the flight, the more expensive it is. Airlines do consider cutting down the routes for more frequent destinations in a day. Reducing the frequencies for short destinations will ensure the availability of the flights for the immediate next short destination. So by focusing on only short-haul flights, a single aircraft can cover several short-haul destinations in a day. Nevertheless, the frequencies will be lesser.

Long haul flights are not cost-efficient because it needs more jet fuels to burn. The demand for long-haul flights needs to be at least 90% to meet the original cost structure for the routes.

When the demand is not steady, it means the revenue generated will not be sufficient to cover the cost all the time. It gives a higher probability of losing money instead of making money. So cutting on the long haul flights and destinations would be wiser to be replaced with connecting routes of several short-haul flights. Having more stops can carry inter-destination passengers. More passengers who are comfortable with one or more stops to reach their destinations. It will be cost-effective and therefore the fare is possibly lesser too.

With all the aspects, the number of flights owned or leased by an airline determines the ultimate debt of the airline. During this pandemic season, having more aircraft in the field could cost so much as not every flight is flying. So taking this opportunity to seize the little possible revenue, cutting down the number of fleets to only those that are flying and will possibly fly for the next few months. The remaining fleets could be returned to the lease company after renegotiating the agreements, and for airlines with parent companies, returning fleets to them would be extremely beneficial in weathering this storm.

Growing smaller is inclusive of having lesser staff, retrenchments and furloughs are the last resort for airlines. In this COVID-19 scenario, none of the airlines could make it without meeting the last resort at least once. It will be a very emotional moment in the headlines and all over social media, yet this situation has to be tackled with a special team. The employees would mourn over but the management of the whole retrenchment process makes the difference in experience. The reality is that airlines are only able to survive when retrenchment happens as it cuts the cost of payrolls. Offering partial pay cuts to the remaining employees and making them feel appreciated with the management gestures. Retrenchment is needed but retaining skilled employees with regular training and certifications is an important aspect not to forget on.

On the other hand, the airlines could grow smaller and more compassionate. The alternative solution would be attrition and a hiring freeze. Attrition morally acts more, it conveys the airlines' compassion towards their existing employees. Attrition is a process of resignation or retirement of employees with their concerns. It is a voluntary process with the employees' comfort and timeline. Employees will be called and informed ahead of the airlines' situation and both the airline and the employee can take the best decision for survival.

Hiring freeze for the positions of employees who have been retrenched or furloughed or went through attrition. Instead of hiring new employees, the airlines could plan to reposition the job description. In this way, the airlines could leverage the existing workforce to minimize overhead costs and as well as minimize workforce loss.

3.5 WAY FORWARD FOR THE SUSTAINABLE AIRLINE INDUSTRY

The airline industry of a certain country is small yet important. The future of the industry is highly associated with the pride of the nation. The growth of the future airline industry is going to be massive as there are a lot of efforts taken to make the airline experience seamless and affordable. The airline industry takes advanced systems and technologies as the frontier of sustainability. Four main aspects of growth in the future airline industry to make justice for sustainability have been identified as technology growth, CORSIA initiatives, big data application, infrastructure improvisations, and most importantly innovative business model.

3.5.1 Technology

The whole process and experience at the airport before departure and arrival need to be very seamless and contactless in the future. Airlines need to invest in super app construction for the passengers as well as for the airlines. The super app will be promising a future of profitability with the digital shift replacing all the traditional experiences of the airline industry. The super app should be an app for bookings, add-on, digital boarding passes with QR codes and add-on services such as food on-board or bundled hotel bookings. The airline has to focus on the technologies to develop biometrics and facial recognition too. This covers the basic necessary items and also leisure items to be sold on the app. Airlines can generate additional revenue by providing this app for collaboration with local vendors to promote and sell their goods and services online too. This app platform works as simple as other online platforms like Alibaba and Lazada which gives a win-win situation for both airlines and vendors. This seizes the opportunity to attract locals to the international platform. On the other hand, airlines benefit by having all the ultimate data of the people's behaviour and offer the best-bundled offer by analyzing every customer's need. In other words, each customer receives a customized unique selling proposition (USP). Meanwhile, the app tackles the main issue of the post-pandemic, offers social distancing, paperless and contactless boarding, and reduces congestion at the airport. The obtained data will be used for airline operations and make it faster and more efficient by leveraging the digital ecosystem. This can be even further developed from a 'walkthrough' experience in the airport to the flights. The facial recognition measures can be enhanced to make it as advanced as it acts as an international passport. This means, a passenger can stand on a designated social distance box in a travellator conveyer mechanism at the entrance of the airport and the travellator moves the passenger through a few facial recognition and scanners for all the screening until the boarding gate. So a passenger does not need to be in contact with anyone or any object when he or she is boarding a plane and the same goes for the arrival too

3.5.2 CORSIA

Throughout the deep pandemic situation, the airline industry has seen the 'greener' industry. This is because due to lesser flights, the emission has been lesser as well. The airline industry has to take this action to provide the best sustainability attention and care. Airlines should change the perspective of the industry to be more efficient by conserving energy and focussing on profitability. The research world needs to pay attention to aid the industry to experience the green technology shift. International Civil Aviation Organization (ICAO) has launched the Carbon Offsetting and Reduction Scheme for International Aviation or well known as CORSIA. This initiative is mainly to achieve carbon-neutral growth from the year 2020. Civil airlines worldwide should join the campaign for clean air. Kerosene is cheaper compared to electro-fuel. This is one of the reasons airlines choose kerosene over other fuels, but it is a highly polluting fuel. To keep growing in the airline industry and expand the number of flights, the usage of kerosene needs to be reduced and the industry shall shift to cleaner fuels. One of the ways is by taxing the kerosene as this will reduce the price gap between kerosene and cleaner fuels. On the other side, the research world needs to continuously work toward the energy-conscious airline industry by producing affordable clean jet fuels for many. This sustainability measure needs to be accompanied by lawmakers. The development of the law for the green industry takes progressive time and can be accelerated with constant monitoring with the industry partners.

3.5.3 Big Data

Big data will be playing the master role in the technology shift. The green industry needs to be achieved as a community of the industry. This initiative can never be done alone. The connective platform between the airlines in the same region at least needs to be paid attention to kick-start the effort. An airline has tonnes of data. These data can be leveraged precisely to manipulate the deviations to promote positive growth for the airlines. However, as advanced the big data analytics could be, it would not be materialized without collaboration with other technologies. The important collaboration would be with other communication satellites and a new generation of high-speed internet connections across the globe. The information retracted from the big data can be used to develop artificial intelligent (AI) humanoids which can make supply chain management seamless. Alongside, the app specialist and the internet of things (IoT) play the platform construction initiatives. Airlines need to adopt and adapt digital technologies to their services as soon as possible to secure a future airline industry. Investments in engineering projects are merely to boost the efficiency of the industry

3.5.4 Infrastructure

As for airlines, local travel is expected to be increasing. People will be moving out internally first before they start flying freely overseas. The local state safety will be visible and convincing more than international safety assurance. Therefore, in near future, local travels are expected to bloom. An increase in the number of passengers simply challenges the two most important aspects, the first would be the air space limitations and the second would be the infrastructure. Expecting an airport to accommodate the social distance criteria means a larger infrastructure which is not the solution. Therefore, need to come out with an alternate efficient way to accommodate the growth by 2024. Infrastructure does not just stop physically, it means the virtual infrastructure too. Virtual infrastructure emphasizes more the app constructions for the one-point contact for passengers, airlines as well as stakeholders. For a million over-data-supported technology to run the industry, a powerful and accommodative virtual infrastructure is the key.

3.5.5 Innovative Business Model

Airlines' survival strength has even pushed the airlines to come up with innovative business models. One of our very own Malaysian low-cost carriers has set the greatest example by exploring newer business models by leveraging their strengths, and digital skills. During the time whereby the whole country stayed in the solitude of curbing COVID-19, the low-cost airline accelerated its pace through digital transformation such as e-hailing rides, food delivery, and e-shop. The airline has managed to breathe throughout the pandemic season and even better in the endemic season.

3.6 CONCLUSION

COVID-19 is a global pandemic that can reshape the airline industry. Flying will be an entirely new experience. COVID-19 is another setback for the airline industry, following 9/11 and the 2008 financial crisis. It has exacerbated the aviation industry's worst crisis in history. The airline industry has never encountered anything remotely comparable to the COVID-19 pandemic. COVID-19 has rewritten the industry's history.

Government intervention is needed to protect the nation and people from the spread of deadly diseases. Governments have taken strict measures of travel restrictions and border closures which have eventually left the airline industry in a dark shell. These two strict rules have hit the airline industry directly as that is what an airline caters for. The business model of the airlines depends on travel and crossing the borders freely.

However, despite the bankruptcies filed by numerous airlines, most of the airlines are still trying to turn around their fate by taking drastic recovery ways. The recovery is supported by local government, investors, and other shareholders. Together the recovery would be faster and more efficient. To have a sustainable airline industry, future research and direction should move towards the advancement of technologies, CORSIA, leveraging big data, focusing on the virtual infrastructure compared to physical infrastructure, and most importantly venture into new business models. COVID-19 might be the first and last deadliest pandemic ever, it might have caused unforeseen damages abruptly, yet this serves as a lesson and better prepares the airline industry for an unbeatable future.

ACKNOWLEDGEMENT

In preparing the book chapter, I am indebted to Dr. Shathees for giving me this golden opportunity to contribute to a book chapter. I would like to thank him for the guidance and for setting a high benchmark for the quality of the write-up. I would like to express my gratitude to Malindo Airways Sdn Bhd for providing me the platform to know in-depth the real situation before I could put my thoughts together in this chapter write-up. Thank you for all the access to the virtual meetings that I have been a part of. This is indeed a proud moment of producing the chapter as this is where my heart and soul always are

REFERENCES

Air Transport Bureau. (2020). Effects of Novel Coronavirus (COVID-19) on Civil Aviation: Economic Impact Analysis. Retrieved October 26, 2020, from https://www.icao.int/sustainability/Pages/Analyses-and-Forecasting.aspx

Choong, J. (2020, June 4). Report: AirAsia to Lay Off 250 Staff Members Following Covid19 Downturn. Retrieved online from https://www.malaymail.com/news/malaysia/2020/06/04/report-airasia-to-lay-off250-staff-members-following-covid-19-downturn/1872493

Fine, D., Klier, J., Mahajan, D., Raabe, N., Schubert, J., Singh, N., & Ungur, S. (2020, April 15). How to Rebuild and Reimagine Jobs Amid the Coronavirus Crisis from https://www.mckinsey.com/industries/public-and-social-sector/our-insights/how-to-rebuild-and-reimagine-jobs-amid-the-coronavirus-crisis

Kaur, D. (2021, February 26). How Airasia Pivoted its Airline Business to Survive a Pandemic from https://techwireasia.com/2021/02/heres-how-airasia-pivoted-its-airline-business-to-survive-the-pandemic/

Kenton, W. (2020b). What Is Attrition?. Retrieved online from https://www.investopedia.com/terms/a/attrition.asp#:~:text=Attrition%20is%20a %20process%20in,and%20reduce%20payroll%20than%20layoffs

Maneenop, S., & Kotcharin, S. (2020). The Impacts Of COVID-19 On The Global Airline Industry: An Event Study Approach. *Journal of Air Transport Management.* Volume 89, October 2020, 101920.

Singh, Padmalini & P, Nuthan & Hung, Yip & Mui, Daisy & Kee, Daisy & Yap, Sing & Pandey, Divya & Pandey, Rudresh & Yunn, Sek & Foo, Shelly & Wen, Hui. (2021). Alternative Strategies to Avoid Layoff in Airlines Industry During the Covid-19 Pandemic.

Subramaniam, S. (2020, September 29). Inside The Airline Industry's Meltdown from

https://www.theguardian.com/world/2020/sep/29/inside-the-airline-industry-meltdown-coronavirus-pandemic

CHAPTER 4

Work-from-Home: Present and Post COVID-19 Work Trends – What's Emerging?

Shatish Rao Samtharam

4.1 INTRODUCTION

The author has started the chapter by highlighting the changes that happened in common work practices during the outbreak of COVID-19 and how do those changes take place. The author also highlighted the implication that can be foreseen while working from home and how will it affect the work-life of individuals. The author has shared some concepts on how individuals can deal with emerging "new norms" in work practices and lastly emphasizes that WFH is a permanent shift in work practices.

4.2 THE CHANGE IN WORK PRACTICES

The focus in recent years has been on digitalization and the Industrial Revolution 4.0. We now live in a rapidly growing environment where changes are often needed in the world of work. Technology has evolved quickly, but is it able to realize this Industrial 4.0, or perhaps is it just a marketing gimmick? (Kathirgugan, 2020). If so, how do the workers benefit from it? Let's see the very real situation in this chapter.

This pandemic has forced a new revolution in work practices which is the 'Work from Home (WFH) concept. If innovations in technology are believed to be beneficial for employees, how many businesses have sought to allow their employees to work from home before?

Web conferencing software that facilitates high-performance video and audio conferencing for internal communication is not something new in the world of the internet. Yet, companies widely believe efficiency is higher with the presence of employees in the workplace. Remote work practice was taken into account since 1984, as employees of the white-collar would be working from anywhere. Unfortunately, this projection did not come to light entirely even after 33 years (Ryan, 2017, quoted from Forbes 2017). Many employers have failed to alter all this while encouraging their workers to function remotely presumed due to mentality, status quo, and entrenched standards. There is much evidence of WFH practice by industries, yet most are reported failures. A renowned brand such as Yahoo and IBM for example has recalled its remote employees back to the office (Ryan, 2017) due to the perceived lack of innovative staff, which is seen as the main strategy of that company (Pathak, Bathini, Kandathil, 2015). Despite technology, even high-profile organizations have pulled their handbrakes to enable remote operations.

Trust is a fundamental issue in this aspect. Most employers have found a lack of confidence in their subordinates or colleagues. They are afraid, instead of trusting. The lack of confidence makes employees commute every day to work so that their superiors can supervise them (Ryan, 2017). Managers want their employees to be in the workplace so that teams can collaborate and work together. When a pandemic such as COVID-19 had spread massively, driving people away from the office, managers struggled because they failed to understand the nature of working remotely.

COVID-19 has shown the world that WFH practices could keep businesses running and sustained. After a declaration of a health emergency in many nations, it took only a few days for companies to allow their employees to work from home.

During the COVID-19 outbreak, the implementation of the WFH guidelines was swift but never smooth as it accounts for a series of issues. WFH seems simple and appealing to employees as they have the bandwidth to stay at home. However, it is very new for many, and they have not been adequately trained. There were no instructions or framework to ensure that outcomes were obtained as expected. The pandemic was unforeseen, and organizations were not prepared for the WFH norm.

Nevertheless, most employees have experienced work from home despite all the hassles, especially the white collars. Generally, these are the employees (for example, accountants, consultants, attorneys, and managers) that enrol on non-routine jobs and hardly do manual labour (AccountingTools, 2021). They also enjoy the freedom of working hours to do their jobs based on the workloads. On top of these, now they have experienced the tips and tricks to make work feasible from home. Some employees saw work from home culture as a perfect fit, but some chose to return to their office to work. Before we got on with the new norm, employees had the option of working from home. It has become a course or a strategy of the organization after the COVID-19 pandemic, but it is still a battle to preserve this new existence.

4.3 A HARD JUMP START FOR WFH PRACTICES

Let's go back further in time. Who used to work from home traditionally? As technology develops, the life of the white-colored occupants is slowly remodelled. Clerical personnel like customer service agents, telemarketers, and people performing repeated tasks "digitally" were encouraged to work from home, predominantly during work shifts. During the days, professional researchers began demanding more flexibility and autonomy than clerical employees with higher wages without bounding to any work hours.

Also, their employers allowed them the opportunity to prepare and deploy their privacy whenever they intend but, they were still required to visit their co-workers if any consultation on the job was needed. This initial stage of white dollars gave companies certain confidence that computer-based employees are suitable employees who can operate from home.

This transition has intensified since the 'Industrial Revolution 4.0' was laid on by the economy and business world. If the industry is championed by artificial intelligence, cloud computing, and big data, the employees need to undergo professional training to handle this intelligence. The world moves forward with the implementation of cyber-physical systems for factories, offices, or even small-scale businesses, while employees improve their digitalization skills in remote management of their smart systems.

As society grows, all types of employees have been affected. From Gen-X to millennials employees, all are getting ready to embrace this new norm. On the other hand, there are employees around us who have trouble adjusting to this transition. By working in their office setting physically, these employees have brought impacts, values, and greater accomplishments to their workplace. They want to be in the office or production lines to make sure it goes hand in hand. Their experience has proven that 'physical presence is the most effective way to move the organization forward. This does not mean that senior employees are not welcomed to operate remotely as most of them have been used from the very beginning to develop their company by engaging with their colleagues or senior employers physically. Before virtual communication systems took place, their jobs went quicker face to face with negotiations, meetings, and decisions. Besides, one-on-one sessions with colleagues have improved their relationships and encouraged sustainable workplace trust.

They typically 'segmented' their professional working life and personal life and did not have them affect each other. This is where they have mastered the Work-Life Balance (WLB) practices.

Therefore, there comes the challenge of adaptation when these employees are required to WFH, especially during the COVID-19 outbreak. Organizations provide the greatest support for their physical and financial survival when it comes to offering smartphones, tablets, and subscriptions to interaction platforms such as Zoom and Teams accounts to ensure that employees work from home. Although it is for a long-term adaptation, organizations also have some concerns (Finnegan, 2020). Poor internet accessibility and limited experience in digital video interaction have created difficulties for them to operate remotely as well.

It was up to the respective organizations to determine before WFH policies became binding law. Occasionally, employees are employed at home voluntarily. Most of the time it happens whenever they have to work to resolve their ad-hoc businesses and handle their inevitable family affairs together.

Sadly, it has never lasted

The way of managing the workforce in a 'working environment' and the ease in the segmentation of work and family time has become close to impossible while working from home. However, when these concepts were taken over by managers or senior managers, their subordinates were expected to function the same way as these seniors. This was giving a hard jumpstart for work-from-home practices.

Not all can work from home all the time. Perhaps everyone will accept work-from-home policies at some point.

The global market was sluggish during the pandemic COVID-19 but I was not irrecoverable. This also refers to the working conditions. It is like a pendulum; it could swing back to the same place. Every company decided to change by working from home, at least for the time being, just to break the chain of COVID-19.

Professional employees that are so used to working at office desks around us have not felt comfortable working from home. Of course, most of them must be on site with the support of their team or colleagues to prepare, deploy, and monitor the work. Therefore, if any of them operate from home, if their colleagues find themselves in some ad-hoc situation, they cannot offer immediate assistance. This can affect both site employees' efficiency.

That is to say, employees' success is not only determined by their abilities and competency, but also by their colleagues who WFH. Some employees have also revealed that the increasing interdependence between colleagues and complexities in many jobs indicates that employees work to achieve the organizational objective as a whole, depending on each other's work. During crises or ad-hoc workplace problems, the employees in charge were required to return to work even though they are scheduled to work at home. After years of working in office cubicles, employees that worked various shifts are scheduled to work remotely. They may be no longer perceive the working 'culture' to which they have adhered for many years. The working culture has changed. They do not have a social bond or reinforce their relationship physically in a team. They are not experiencing the gist exchange of ideas as they work together as well.

As a result, the value of the business and team culture dramatically changed.

Indefinitely, is working from home safer than conventional work methods? Let us now go a little backward and refresh how many years we've been in the past.

The typical working hours for all employees working in the offices is nine to ten hours per day. Commonly, employees of course particularly snoozing once hated the agony of their morning alarm. After a couple of tough minutes, force themselves to dress in their casual clothes, get a little coffee, prepare breakfast for themselves and their families, and send their children to school.

Those driving to work regularly are still on the road to their survival in high-speed traffic time, and the blood-sucking parking payment and lift as they are needed on time at work. How about those who rely on public transportation, on the other hand? For many people, it has never been easy to manage individual time with transport services timing. Some spend more time travelling from their homes to workplaces. One's job could be far away from their office. So, they choose to wake up earlier than those who have cars or motorbikes to prevent further complications. It does not stop here, there are thousands of people in a day riding public transport such as trains or buses. The crowds will cause inconvenience for the users during peak hours. By enduring all the problems, these classes of employees still have no privilege to start work late, nor do the management or human resources policies accept their difficulties.

During working hours, employees must push through all of the constants banters, politics, bickering, and even amusing lame jokes to face each other are everyday norms. Furthermore, these employees relentlessly brickbat their points with certain annoying HR rules to stick to. Also, during chain breaks, they have to hang out together for lunches in the closest cafeterias, cafes, or food courts for a few minutes before the break-outs. All are part of the whole working journey.

Traditionally, employees have dreaded Mondays to Thursdays, been terrified of working late in the office, and whine about an unfair schedule all week long. 'Thank God it's Friday' is what they celebrated after a week of everlasting meetings and distracting employers' sermons. They feel like they're not paid slaves anymore at this moment and have freedom for the rest of the week.

All these were routine until COVID-19 strikes.

Instantly, there is no trouble in commuting to work, running for lunches, or going to meeting rooms. Simultaneously, no set period is available for employees to work, whether on a Monday or Sunday. No lazy weekends or a savage getaway to rest and chill out. In the new work atmosphere, which is their home, they are not given a fixed time to take lunch or coffee breaks.

4.4 IS IT GOODBYE FOR OFFICE CUBICLES?

It often involves working together with people from diverse backgrounds, perceptions, behaviours, and attitudes in a specific building or room to carry out the required work in support of the organization's mission and vision. However, after the coronavirus pandemic, the exacerbating employees were worried about returning to their office spaces (Gibbens, 2020).

Not everyone will stay and work at home. Such individuals will also go to their offices based on their line of work and orders. On normal days, certain workplaces appeared intrusive and distractive. Today, with those returning to their workplace, they might feel that through this pandemic the possible health threat is still around them. Corporations hardly alter the plans of the office floor. When the offices reopened, people's well-being was still at stake. Many companies recruit suppliers to disinfect the entire workstation, however, the original arrangement of the work areas and the gaps between working tables or cubicles (for example), remain the same which creates unavoidable concerns among employees.

Working coworkers had the opportunity to select their desks before the new standard came into practice. If someone does not like his cubicle mate, there were other cubicles for them to change to. Some people may enjoy talking, so they prefer to work in a position packed with close colleagues. But now employees need to be a little distant from their peers for physical isolation and infection prevention.

Spacious workplace layouts are a deterrent to the spread of this virus from one to another. When someone is sick but not yet tested, it will potentially infect others if physical touches, sneezes, or toughs are not maintained properly. Some surfaces such as a door handle or tables are often used to transmit this disease to co-workers.

With fixed office layouts, employers and human resources should consider alternatives such as staggered employee arrival times, directing office foot traffics, and staging areas for the elevator. Furthermore, it would be beneficial to minimize the number of chairs for face-to-face sessions, reduce the number of seats in lounges, build standardized corridors with social distance and issue recommendations for the physical removal of the office staff.

Having an office could be still a must for any organization but: in a way, it's still can work by preventing the spread and also making offices a healthier place to work.

4.5 WORK-LIFE AFTER COVID-19

With rising technology, well before COVID-19, the world shifted more rapidly. Now the pandemic has just speeded up this process. Organizations now tweak their technology and ability to work, reinvent their workplace, and lead more than ever. Now is the future of jobs.

A shift from "Hard Skills to Soft Skills"

Over the years, companies have prioritized the option of skills to work, read, calculate, and tech skills. Often considered were the traditional soft skills, but not required by the employers anymore. Most individuals will be decently fine as long as the work is done. Today, the expectation of soft skills has changed. They are now autonomous, so during this pandemic, periods of tension, stress, and tragedy, employees should have certain soft skills. According to Morgon (2020), these soft skills are the latest hard skills

Organizations want their employees to be as engaged and corporate as they were in the workplace, and these soft skills are all important. Now employees do not meet physically to explore and communicate the processes of planning. This is the moment where empathy and time management capabilities are established as they report from home. Such skills will sustain their teamwork, their dedication, their zeal, and their momentum and will also influence their colleagues' success.

Flexible management in setting "hours & location"

People wanted employment and work to be paid for and to provide permanent job security. To sustain the objective, people must have adequate versatility, especially with their position and time. Each of the personal rooms in the houses of employees may be turned into a bed and work during regular work or closing periods respectively. It depends on the essence of the company and these are usually the way to operate from home.

Job and family life are managed by people, so colleagues and supervisors should understand and embrace sessions or consultations during non-working hours. It does not stop there. The location places an enormous part to have unrestricted meetings by Zoom. Hence, employees should know which the most suitable place is to pick for their meeting.

"New coaching & mentoring methods"

Managers must not dictate what to do, but they must begin to see their role as the creation of other leaders. Each employee operates individually with limited supervision, so today's leaders need to be a lighthouse for success and sustainability.

They must consistently expand on their duty to inspire, empower, and supervise employees by utilizing telecommunications and immersive training to establish autonomous leaders and lead their work.

From "working like robots" to "working with AI and robots"

This is an employees' frequent concern. They ought to show themselves at once in the workplace, wear the same clothing, do the same job, eat, and leave home simultaneously. This is customary for daily employees who have made them look like a robot. Before robot inventions exist, people are the best option for work, but now the world has technologies that can execute robotic functions.

So, then how about humans?

People need not go against these innovations to thrive, but they have to improve their imagination and strategic facets of work by using these robots and Ai(s). These things do not necessitate people being on the job. They just have the systems from home to power.

From "Process-centric" to "Strategic-focused" tasks

A process-based job entails joining pieces of puzzles in transfer work, but strategic-based concentrates more on solving a challenge or problem. When focusing on collaborating with AI, robotics, and independent leaders, people must begin to unleash their capacity to do things in an innovative, special, problem-solving way, and to conceive about the broader picture to move things as quickly as possible. Not that it is not good to be process-centered, but that it needs better coordination and comprehension. Although automation is to bring employees to work together it prohibits employees from going independently. It does not just work 'your' jobs in a process, but people need to know 'how' and 'where' the method operates.

From "Hierarchy-structured" to "Flatter-structured"

For decades, employers have monitored their employees from their vision and discouraged them, due to their so-called seniority rank, from speaking out their opinion. The employees want their voices to be heard even when they were isolated from their jobs physically. It would further obstruct their concerns by placing hierarchy systems and separating them emotionally from operational facets. Telecommunication is already a successful forum and businesses still can be utilizing it further to break the pyramid rule and flatten it.

It's not only about "Job", but now it's about "Job and Life"

People work, but no longer in the workplace. They work in their homes with their children or parents. Therefore, things such as life quality, intent, and importance are now what employees expect most, just as they must. Employees did not ask for the experience of a pandemic or life after a pandemic. That is what employees experience and it's a game-changer.

The aim should be to help the organization and the people who contribute to sustainability as well. To do this, businesses must pick up work from home practices and work closely on budget strategies, operating practices, and strategic plans that will lead to the well-being of their employees.

From "pen and paper" to "digitalize everything"

The COVID-19 pushed several organizations, using new networks and technology, to force their workers to operate remotely from home. Many companies spoke of Industrial Revolution 4.0 but some were very hesitant before COVID-19 to introduce WFH policies. One of the principal factors, whether they believed it or not, was that most companies still lack digital transformation.

They have no alternative during the COVID-19 outbreak. People had to practice social distancing. In several countries, work from home has been a mandate. Thus, solutions were considered as mechanisms of digitalization, telecommunications, and interactive collaboration. All have been automated to enhance teamwork and execution. Manual procedures such as the signing of papers, paper printing for meetings, and even processes relating to the implementation of work could be digitalized to enable work to be virtually progressed without any direct meetings.

From "work-life balance" to "work-life integration"

Last but not the least, work from home (WFH), as mentioned, it is a game-changer that changed the way people approach their work and their family boundaries. The working day is 9-5 so what happens before 9-5 is purely personal time. However, during this period people would be able to work and still carry out their family duties.

There has been a boundary between home and job for many years. It was a personal life after work. It's all about jobs after home. There is a huge change here. Today, it's a change of juggling life and employment from managing life after work, where workers are living and working. It's a norm today.

4.6 THE EMERGENCE OF WORK-LIFE INTEGRATION

Speaking of work and life, the way of living and working has changed. For many years people were talking about the heights of work-life balance (WLB). It was the best to equally excel and balance time with work, family, friends, and personal interests.

The distinctions between work and life are required for people to differentiate. People are ambitious in dichotomizing all lives, but analysts argue that this concept leads to confusion and dilemmas when work reaches home (Delanoeije, Verbruggen, & Germeys, 2019; Bhumika, 2020).

Yes, it is creating artificial segregation between life and work as IF work is not a part of life (Cheng-Tozun, 2018).

In the case of life losses when operating, even some say, WLB will not follow the zero-sum equation and vice versa. In contrast, the hours spent at home, given the hours spent working for the family, also causes burnout. Employees ended up overworking at home and hurting their social or non-work life, which unfortunately led to unhappiness all around (Clark, 2021).

Many, especially working from home parents have faced a lot of challenges to get through their workday without interruptions, in particular, the ones with kids. Beyond just fulfilling the childcare demands, parents are in a situation to fill other roles, such as being homeschool teachers. Supervising and assisting their kids in online education while managing work matters is surely not an easy task to do during remote work (Stahl, 2022). On top of it, they are also playing the role of homemaker for their family while focusing on daily workloads. Apart from being in a parenting role, they are expected to be in a position of a helpful spouse and the one who gets necessary groceries as well. At times, working parents smears into a long-chained streak of discussions and meetings where there might be no stopping points. Not everyone can be good at multi-tasking and dividing their focus between work and family. It is a real challenge to switch modes and find times in both domains (Durand, 2020).

Hence, in this case, it is practical to say work-life balance is impossible to happen during working from home (Prasad, 2017)

An idea called the integration of working and life has been implemented in the last few years and has become increasingly popular. However how many people know that precisely, and how useful it can be?

UC Berkeley's Haas School of Business reports work-life integration is an approach to creating greater synergy between all fields, describing 'life' that integrates 'home, work, culture, health, and personal well-being.' It provides the freedom to cross borders and meshes perfectly with daily life for people with both work and family commitments (Cheng-Tozun, 2018).

A standard work-life Integration would opt to have breakfast with his/her family and then drop the children in school and then start work from nine to 1 p.m. then go to work after lunch and have lunch, then have to take the children from school to cook dinner for them and reply to the outstanding emails till the bedtime.

To juggle work, elderly parents, spouse, kids, house works, and hobbies, Work-Life Integration will be the ideal way to have and do it all. It is a solution for minimizing employee disputes. It remains debatable, though since the answer would not be optimal for everybody.

If workers or even entrepreneurs become endless with their to-do list, they can feel compelled to fill every couple of inches of their lives with working time, without giving health, families, and society the same priority. When this occurs, the work integrates itself very much into all aspects of life without introducing a lot of life into the day. This causes them to constantly think about their work only even though initiatives are taken to pay attention to other priorities.

What leads to it?

For many, job obligations seem to take precedence over our loved ones' or our day-to-day needs. Once we are motivated by obligations and their urgencies, we shall reflect first of all on these stresses. If we all pay attention to our work first it will never be possible.

How to avoid this and make work-life Integration truly work for us?

Make schedules: discipline and reverence in every timetable, including in integration. All on the schedule should be. It may sound formal, but it tells you in certain respects "what to manage in which time." Both the schedules should be structured in such a way as to attend events, prepare for family meals, night jogs, or run activities.

Coordination: It is good to have plans, but while you are with your spouse or family it is important to plan them and it demonstrates that you prioritize your family when focusing on jobs on the other hand.

Boundary commitments: work is limitless, so there is no problem disconnecting it to allow you some rest. Give yourself a few days or weeks to stop worrying about work and concentrate on your people and your favourite things.

Our lives must be strongly packed with valuable work and relationships. The convergence of work and life should be made simpler and richer for both. It does not come easily. It needs practice, prioritization, and execution.

4.7 WORK FROM HOME: IT IS HERE TO STAY

Many have considered whether they want to continue operating from home after the COVID-19 lockdown. Employers and administrations have already coerced WFH staff but will have the right to request them in the future.

It is proven, that WFH is workable.

Some thought this WFH would be a temporary transition, but the WFH idea is alive and safer than ever as time goes on. Group investments in office or design layouts and technology on the premises are being limited. This cost reduction is not only for companies but also for the employees. They do not have to drive, buy food for lunch, and other varied expenses. The best part is that these financial advantages come with minimum disruption to employees' productivity levels and their wellbeing.

Nor is this over soon, nor will it last long. People need to hope that there will be a future in which COVID-19 cases stopped spreading one day and life recovers steadily. However, in between people with entire organizations will be transformed to survive and succeed. And, in the context of WFH policies, it needs support. Since this worldwide pandemic, several nations are already operating from home. Every organization has its way of operating, so each one must define it for the workers' comparison in particular. Following Covid-19, individuals will be allowed to return to work, but not all are called at a time. Some can use a hybrid strategy, where more than 2 employee groups can work remotely on alternative days or weeks. Again, it depends on the industry and business nature. The SOPs must be reported in proper WFH policy to ensure a realistic culture of the workplace without disrupting processes or employee productivity when work is performed with dispersed teams.

After we won COVID-19, companies will have well-evolved WFH policies for the long term with what they have experienced and learned throughout the process.

Management of human capital is an important aspect of this. They need to have their employees with them, progress continues but without getting burned out. It's not easy, but it's not impossible as well. Besides the regulations, businesses require simulated training on WFH policies, technologies and IT growth, and work-life boundary management, who are concerned to improve their employees. The world has evolved, and the employees should also comply. To do so, they also need to have a review mechanism on employees regarding their experience while working from home. Organizations should have a flatter system of leadership so that employees can articulate their complaints about the gap. To track employees' current understanding of WFH, a review process of the WFH is required.

WFH is not just a solution during pandemics, in a way it demonstrates concern, interest, and career opportunities and creates trust so that businesses can begin to respond to any phenomenon.

4.8 CONCLUSION

COVID-19 has entirely reshaped "the future of work". It was not an easy journey or a simple beginning. WFH has both benefits and drawbacks. It was a challenge, for those who never worked remotely but it was a bonus for companies to keep alive. The result is that it's going to work; however, time is needed. All have diverse experiences with which it is too difficult to incorporate.

This is the emerging working autonomous model. The concern is not how to embrace it nor how we can function independently. The pandemic COVID-19 has changed employees' careers and lives. Work from Home (WFH) will begin to evolve with the existence of digitalization. It is now up to your hands to be free to follow this new standard or to become chaotic, by being reluctant to adopt it in the future.

ACKNOWLEDGEMENT

Writing this chapter was harder than I thought and more appreciating than I have imagined. All this would not be possible without Dr. Shathees, the soul behind turning an idea into a book. Thank you for trusting me and making things possible.

A very special thanks to Mrs. Tejasvini Shanmuganathan as well, for reading the early drafts of this chapter to offering the best advice on the writing so I can deliver the best. She was important to this chapter getting done as well. Thank you so much.

REFERENCES

AccountingTools. (2021, December 23). *White Collar Worker Definition*. Retrieved from https://www.accountingtools.com/articles/white-collar-worker.

Allenby, B., & Fink, J. (2000). Social and ecological resilience: Toward inherently secure and resilient societies. *Science, 24*(3), 347-64.

Bhumika, (2020). Challenges for Work-life Balance during COVID-19 Induced Nationwide Lockdown: Exploring Gender Difference in Emotional Exhaustion in the Indian Setting. *Gender In Management, Ahead-of-print (Ahead-of-print)*. https://doi.org/10.1108/GM-06-2020-0163.

Cheng-Tozun, D. (2018, March 14*). Work-Life Balance vs. Work-Life Integration: How Are They Different, and Which One Is for You?*. Retrieved from https://www.inc.com/dorcas-cheng-tozun/how-work-life-integration-can-help-you-have-it-all.html.

Clark, A. (2021, July 22). 5 *Common Problems Plaguing Remote Workers and What to do About Them*. Retrieved from https://www.forbes.com/sites/forbesbusinesscouncil/2021/07/22/5-common-problems-plaguing-remote-workers-and-what-to-do-about-them/?sh=4cfda9c4c57f.

Delanoeije, J., Verbruggen, M., & Germeys, L. (2019). Boundary Role Transitions: A Day-to-day Approach to Explain the Effects of Home-based Telework on Work-to-home Conflict and Home-to-work Conflict. *Human Relations, 72*(12), 1843-1868.

Finnegan, M. (2020, October 5). *Working From Home? Slow Broadband, Remote Security Remain Top Issues.* Retrieved from https://www.computerworld.com/article/3584454/working-from-home-slow-broadband-remote-security-remain-top-issues.html.

Gibbens, S. (2020, April 30). *Goodbye to open office spaces? How experts are rethinking the workplace.* Retrieved, from https://www.nationalgeographic.com/science/2020/04/will-coronavirus-end-the-open-office-floor-plan/.

ILO. (2020, April 07). *COVID-19 causes devastating losses in working hours and employment.* Retrieved November 10, 2020, from https://www.ilo.org/global/about-the-lo/newsroom/news/WCMS_740893/lang--en/index.htm.

Kathirgugan, K. (2020, October 06). *Is Industry 4.0 (IR 4.0) a gimmick?.* Retrieved from https://www.freemalaysiatoday.com/category/opinion/2020/10/06/is-industry-4-0-ir-4-0-a-gimmick/.

Pathak, A. A., Bathini, D. R. & Kandathil, G. M., (2015). The Ban on Working from Home Makes Sense for Yahoo. It needs the Innovation and Speed of Delivery that Come from Office-based Employees. *Human Resource Management International Digest, 23*(3), 12-14.

Prasad, J. V. (2017). Ignored Aspect of Personal Life in Work-Life Integration. *IOSR Journal of Business and Management, 19*(3), 67-71.

Ryan, L. (2017, March 27). *The Real Reason You're Not Allowed To Work From Home.* Retrieved from https://www.forbes.com/sites/lizryan/2017/03/15/the-real-reason-youre-not-allowed-to-work-from-home/.

Stahl, A. (2021, April 2). *Struggles for Working Parents are Likely to Remain Post-Pandemic.* Retrieved from https://www.forbes.com/sites/ashleystahl/2021/04/02/struggles-for-working-parents-are-likely-to-remain-post-pandemic/?sh=6cd840e26856.

Durand, F. (2020, December 30). *Cooking while Working from Home is Harder than it sounds.* Here's What Works for Me. Retrieved from https://www.thekitchn.com/cooking-ideas-working-from-home-23021122

CHAPTER 5

e-Hailing: Keep Spinning, Wheels

Priyaa Tharisiny Aruldass

5.1 INTRODUCTION

In this chapter, the author discusses the impact of the Covid-19 pandemic on the e-Hailing sector. The author has also included suggestions for future pandemic recovery action. The flow of this chapter is as follows; the chapter started with a brief background study of the e-Hailing sector. This was followed by the impacts of the covid-19 on the e-haling sector worldwide. This leads to the next section of the chapter, whereby the author has discussed the various methods taken by the e-Hailing sector to keep its business afloat amid the deadly pandemic. Lastly, the author has concluded the chapter with suggestions for the future pandemic recovery action plan.

Unexpectedly, a gruesome pandemic has hit our globe in November 2019, causing the spinning world to come to a halt. By day, the virus has spread to all nooks and crooks of the world, creating difficulties for people and causing deaths. COVID-19 pandemic is the greatest communicable disease outbreak to have hit Malaysia since the 1918 Spanish Flu which killed 34,644 people or 1% of the population of the then British Malaya (Hashim, J. H., et al, 2021). Businesses were suspended or shut down altogether, people were forced to stay at home, police forces and army forces have started guarding the streets and the country borders were being closed. Equally importantly, working adults were being retrenched or going on long unpaid leaves. Poverty was rising, it was massive chaos.

In this chaos, many industries face major hits regardless of the country. E-hailing companies faced a slam too. E-Hailing companies are businesses that leverage online applications on smartphones to transport passengers. E-Hailing applications on smartphones can assist customers in performing the following tasks;

- Locate nearby taxis available;
- Allow drivers to identify passengers who require taxi services;
- Book a taxi ride;
- Allow drivers to receive taxi bookings; and
- Make payments online (Horsu & Yeboah, 2015).

The idea of the ride-sharing company started back in the year the 1990s. Before that, people around the world might not have even imagined the possibility of hailing a cab ride with just a touch on their phone screens. The public need to physically walk to the roadside and hail a passing cab or a resting cabbie to get from point A to point B. It was further harder on rainy days.

Gradually, cab bookings via customer service centers were introduced where customers can call the cab service company and schedule a pickup appointment. Later on, when the internet started to progress, new possibilities arose. From there, e-Hailing or formerly known as ride-sharing applications was developed. In the year 2020, commonly heard e-Hailing applications around the world are as the following:

- Uber, Lyft (originated in the United States of America)
- GrabTaxi (originated in Singapore)
- JomRides, Mula (originated in Malaysia)
- Easy Taxi (originated in Brazil)
- Careem (a subsidiary of Uber, based in Dubai)
- Gojek (originated in Indonesia)
- Ola Cabs (originated in India)
- Yandex Taxis (originated in Russia)
- Kakao Taxi (originated in Korea)
- Taxify (now called Bolt, originated in Estonia)

Customers will book a ride via the online application and the payment method would be either cash or cashless. With the emergence of e-Hailing applications, convenience and comfort became a choice and affordable. Initially, cab businesses were thriving in the sector of transporting people. However, as technology advances, individuals came up with the idea of creating online platforms to commute people and eventually add other services such as food and goods delivery. Currently, most of the giant e-Hailing companies have also included food delivery and goods delivery market segments as a part of their portfolio. In this chapter, food delivery and goods delivery services will be treated as a part of services provided by e-Hailing companies and a source of its revenue too. The drivers are usually referred to as driver-partners, while the motorcycle riders who deliver food and goods are usually referred to as delivery partners.

There are many reasons why the setup of e-Hailing platforms was encouraged by the people. The limitation of public transportation services such as buses and minivans in many areas of our globe could be one of the major reasons. The reliability of bus travel schedules is still questionable in many places. With e-Hailing applications, customers can book a ride whenever they are ready to travel. Secondly, the fare for cabs could be on the higher side too. There is no fixed calculation or transparency on the fare imposed, even though there seem to be taxi meters in most cabs. The same 10-kilometer ride could be charged differently by different cab drivers. Moreover, the fare requested at the end of the ride might end up being different than what was initially agreed before the trip because there is no standardization over it. This has increased the frustrations of the users. For e-Hailing applications, this would not be a scenario as the fare is informed to the passengers and drivers before their bookings and it will be fixed unless there is a change in their destinations midway.

Thirdly, the reliability and safety of rides have also improved since the introduction of e-Hailing platforms as both the driver and the passengers are better informed on the lead time taken to reach the destination, the background of the parties involved, and the possibility to share the ride details to loved ones via the applications itself. This has especially become the most favourite feature of women passengers as they can send the ride details to their family or friends and get them to track it. They are assured that if the ride takes longer than necessary or the ride gets disconnected at the wrong drop-off location, somebody will quickly check on them and trigger the police if no response was attained from the passenger.

One of the limiting factors of an e-Hailing application is the necessity to have internet connectivity. It is impossible to hail an e-Hailing car without an internet connection. Therefore, when the phone battery finishes or if a user just got off in a foreign country, customers have no choice but to hail a regular cab or find any other method of transportation.

The main source of revenue for e-Hailing companies comes from car rides because car rides cover the most distance. The idea is simple, a certain percentage of commission is deducted from every car ride. For services such as food delivery and good delivery, a similar calculation applies, however, food delivery services and goods delivery services are usually ordered only within short distances.

On the surface level, it might look as if the driving force of an e-Hailing company is the driver-partners and delivery partners who are on the road, who are getting the work done. However, another equally important driving force is a huge team of dedicated employees who work tirelessly to keep the business going. In an e-Hailing company's organizational structure, the departments in it are very much similar to any other transportation company. The divisions in the departments are usually as the following:

- Sales department
- Human resources department
- Customer service department
- Finance department
- Information technology department
- Marketing department

- Public relations department
- Project management department

The number of employees in an e-Hailing company increases as the company expands its operations to different states and countries.

5.2 IMPACTS OF COVID-19 PANDEMIC ON THE E-HAILING SECTOR

The covid-19 pandemic has hit the e-Hailing sector in a variety of ways. However, not all impacts have been adverse. This section will discuss the adverse impacts and positive impacts of the Covid-19 pandemic on the e-Hailing sector.

5.2.1 Adverse Impacts on the e-Hailing Sector

Alike other industries, the adverse impacts on the e-Hailing sector were evident and undeniable.

Major Drop in Car Ride Bookings

For e-Hailing companies around the world, tourists are the main customers of car rides, and people who commute to work every day come second. Airport rides are commented as one of the most soughed and highest paying rides in this business. With the nation's borders being closed and tourism activities halted, the main source of customers is cut down. According to recent research, the government of Malaysia has recorded losses in tourism of as much as RM 3.37 billion within the first two months of the year 2020 (Karim, W., et al, 2020). It is also reported that travel and tour packages are canceled which affects mostly the hotels and airlines (Aldaihani & Ali, 2018).

Secondly, with employees being forced to work from home, the second source of customers, which are the commuting employees are cut down as well. This leaves little to no customers getting on an e-Hailing ride. In a study published by Statista Research Department, May 26, 2020, 45% of Singaporeans have spent less on ride-Hailing services in April 2020, with a total number of respondents of 2,094. This has directly impacted the revenue of e-Hailing companies.

In Malaysia, the largest e-Hailing company in the year 2020 is GrabTaxi, followed by other popular platforms such as MyCar, Mula, EzCab, and Ryde. The demand for the e-Hailing sector started to see a decrease in January 2020, following the outbreak of Covid-19 in Wuhan, China in November 2019. However, the major blow came when a complete lockdown was imposed on 18th March 2020 throughout the nation. Since the e-Hailing business is categorized as an essential service, the government allowed e-Hailing companies to operate as per usual. However, with limited passengers to carry, e-Hailing companies had to switch their main income from car ride bookings to food deliveries, which only generates barely a quarter of the revenue received from the car rides.

On the other hand, being a highly populated country, Jakarta, Indonesia's capital city has a high number of motorcycle e-Hailing services. Out of many e-Hailing companies, Gojek is the largest player in the industry in 2020. However, with the surge of Covid-19 cases, Gojek has completely got its motorcycle taxi-hailing service deactivated, allowing only food and good delivery services. This has impacted the company's revenue, however, it is impossible to practice social distancing on motorcycle rides. Therefore, they had no choice but to resort to this decision.

High Supply of Driver-Partners Yet Low Demand

When the car ride demands had a sudden drop, the supply becomes high. This increases the fare charges and also creates unhealthy competition among driver-partners. With what few ride bookings available, many drivers' daily income dropped from three digits to as low as one digit.

Increase in Food Delivery Demands, but Low Delivery Partners' Supply

With the surge of home-bounded citizens, food delivery applications became extremely popular. However, as this increase came unnoticed, e-Hailing companies were unprepared. The delivery jobs piled up while there were not enough riders on a platform to cater to them. This has added to a longer waiting time for customers. Naturally, this would induce customers to move to other similar applications since directly walking into restaurants is not an option to buy food for many.

Increase in Operating Cost

e-Hailing drivers are directly in-contact with passengers. They onboard passengers into their personal or hired cars and get them to their destination. With the emergence of new norms such as social distancing, mask adorning, and regular sanitizing, the operating cost of the business increases. Considering safety and health as the most important things at the moment, in many countries, the government has imposed many regulations in response to rising Covid-19 cases such as drivers' cars should be sanitized several times per week and drivers who transport Covid-19 patients must undergo Covid-19 swab tests. Certain companies subsidize these costs as a part of their well-being initiative for their driver-partners. On the other hand, the office buildings of e-Hailing companies among other companies undergo regular sanitization and disinfection. These steps incur the cost. e-Hailing companies have no choice but to follow these regulations imposed by governments to keep operating.

The Emergence of New Players in the Market

Looking at the increasing demand for e-Hailing food delivery services and goods delivery services, many new applications emerge. Besides, individual self-food-delivery businesses were seen a rise too. Many people especially the retrenched working adults turn to home-cooked food delivery businesses to support themselves. They promote their businesses and take orders simply via social media such as WhatsApp, Instagram, and Facebook and deliver them with private vehicles. This has bypassed the conventional system of food ordering via applications and the method continues to grow due to word-of-mouth marketing.

On the other hand, airline businesses started to show interest in airline food delivery services and goods delivery services. Singapore Airlines (SIA) is an example of an airline company that converted its business model to airline meal delivery right to its customers' doorsteps. On October 5th, 2020, SIA received its first airline meal orders from Singaporeans. Besides, in Malaysia, AirAsia launched its first food delivery application named AirAsia Food, which became viral when its CEO Tony Fernandes announced that he will be delivering food orders made upon the application.

The Increased Popularity of Cooking Channels on Social Media

Celebrities and social media influencers around the world have a huge fan base. When this demography started YouTube cooking channels or publish Instagram posts on recipes, their followers tend to embark on making it. With celebrities too being locked in homes and starting cooking channels, their action has increased the interest in people to start cooking their meals. Moreover, the existing cooking channels and celebrity chef channels gain higher popularity amid Covid-19 as well. This has become an indirect threat to e-Hailing delivery businesses as more people have started eating home-cooked meals.

The Sudden Increase in Platform Abuse Cases

In regards to the decrease in car rides, the emergence of modified applications that disrupts the normal framework of the ride allocations and channel the bookings to a specific group of drivers was observed too. These drivers practically steal the rides by bypassing the system. This creates a monopoly of rides and even lesser income for the common drivers who do not use the modified applications. e-Hailing companies such as GrabTaxi and Gojek have given press statements about this and declared this behavior as "fraud".

Besides, an increase in fraud cases on food delivery platforms was observed too, where the number of refund requests by customers multiplied. The refund requests may consist of both valid reasons and invalid reasons. Valid reasons are such as the food packet got broken or drinks spilled during the delivery while invalid reasons could simply be customers' complaints about not receiving some of their ordered items even though they have received them. It is hard to distinguish between valid and invalid reasons, which encourages customers to keep requesting refunds. In August 2020, a 17-year old boy in Singapore has been arrested for the reason of making false refund claims and cheating a food delivery application up to SG$ 14,000.

5.2.2 Positive Impacts on the e-Hailing Sector

There is a proverbial saying that goes "every cloud has a silver lining", which notions no matter how bad a situation goes, there are always some good things that come out of it. This proverbial saying is accurate for the e-Hailing industry because even though the main revenue has been cut off and much firefighting has to be done, some positive impacts and opportunities arose too.

Increases Market Opportunity to Diversify Business

Covid-19 causes people to stay at home, be it working adults, college students, housewives, househusbands, children, and elderly people. With the lockdown situation, people who suffer the most from mealtime is the one that does not know how to cook or those without the facility to cook. Lunchtime became the most important routine of the day, a time off from work or study. This has caused many to turn to food delivery applications to order food online at the click of a screen and get it delivered to their doorsteps. Research published by Statista Research Department on May 26, 2020, shows that about 50% of consumers in Singapore have downloaded a food delivery app during the pandemic. This proves that a new market opportunity has arisen, where ride-hailing companies can leverage their online platforms to start delivering food or increase the number of delivery partners in existing food delivery platforms.

Promotes Word-Of-Mouth Marketing

Since food delivery and good delivery services become a hit among consumers, people tend to share the best experiences they have with a particular brand. This indirectly promotes other consumers to try out the application mentioned too. This is called word-of-mouth marketing and word-out-mouth marketing is by far the best type of traditional marketing in any industry.

Increases Brand Image

During the difficult times of the pandemic, the e-Hailing sector has been identified as one of the essential services among other sectors such as the healthcare sector and banking sector. The delivery partners and driver-partners are being called the esteemed "front-liners", who brave the pandemic and continue to do their jobs despite many challenges faced. This has directly increased the brand image. It has also contributed to the increase in employee satisfaction and loyalty as now the delivery partners and driver-partners are proud to be out there and serving the nation in their way, supporting the government's rules.

Increases Job Opportunities

It is an undeniable fact that many working adults have been retrenched or laid off due to the Covid-19 pandemic. This is one of the ways for a sinking company to stay afloat, is by cutting down the headcounts. Amid this chaos, the e-Hailing food delivery industry strives and provides job opportunities for many out there. In an interview with the regional head of operations for GrabTaxi, Russell Cohen reported that the platform saw a rise in new driver requests, mostly from those who have been laid off. This platform has also become popular among merchants who are looking for ways to promote their businesses and survive financially.

5.3 MEASURES TAKEN BY THE E-HAILING SECTOR TO STAY AFLOAT

To survive in the harsh condition, e-Hailing companies generally looked into several aspects of their operation to firefight. Below listed the measures taken towards different aspects of the business.

5.3.1 Product Diversification and Revenue Management

Like any business, e-Hailing companies around the world tried to stay afloat during this pandemic and also to general revenue. Diversification is the key element of a sustainable business. When the e-Hailing ride demands went down, one of the ways commonly implemented by e-Hailing companies was to onboard more food delivery partners and good delivery partners to cater to the growing demand for these services instead. In Malaysia, GrabTaxi specifically converted drivers to deliver food and goods using their cars instead. This step was largely welcomed as more than thousands of drivers around the nation, especially in Klang Valley started taking up food delivery jobs via their cars. An interview given by Grab's regional head of operations, Russell Cohen revealed that in Malaysia, 18,000 drivers onboarded into food delivery and goods delivery platform within a single day. Gojek, an Indonesia-based start-up application has widened its reach to Vietnam, promoting local SMEs to onboard into its digital platform. They have helped to promote job opportunities among local citizens during the pandemic and helped to increase their market visibility.

Many delivery applications also started providing grocery shopping options where customers can purchase groceries from their favorite marts and get them delivered straight to their doorsteps. Before the pandemic, this idea might not have been largely welcomed by the public as many of the target group are working adults and they rarely be home to receive the goods. They might also have preferred walking directly into the marts at their convenient time and purchasing needed groceries. With most of the working adults forced to work from home, going out seemed like a hassle instead. Not forgetting to mention the risk of attaining or spreading the coronavirus while at shops and marts.

For the Muslims in Malaysia, the holy month of Ramadhan fell during the lockdown period (April-May 2020) imposed by the government. It is a yearly culture where during the Ramadhan month, many people will open up roadside stalls, selling food, drinks, delicacies, and many more. Ramadhan stalls are always heavily crowded and this scenario will last for 1 month. However, in June 2020, the idea of setting up roadside stalls and welcoming huge crowds sounded extremely unsafe. Therefore, the government banned this activity. Looking at this window of opportunity, GrabTaxi introduced E-Kitchen, which allows Ramadhan stall owners to sell their food on Grab App. In collaboration with local government bodies, these Ramadhan stall owners were stationed in several public halls in several states, segregated to avoid overcrowding, and riders or drivers would walk in to pick up the items ordered via the app and get them delivered to customers' delivery locations. This effort boosted both the company revenue and the livelihood of stall owners who only depend on the month of Ramadhan to open their stalls and get the foods and drinks sold.

5.3.2 Managing Headcounts

As listed earlier, an e-Hailing company would have hundreds of employees working for them in different departments, depending on the size of the company. With the sudden drop in its revenue, many e-Hailing companies were pushed to the brink of employee retrenchment. In May 2020, Uber has laid off 3,700 employees to stay in business. While its rival Lyft followed suit and laid off its employees too. Many companies also implemented pay cuts for their higher management staff. On the other hand, portfolio reshuffling was also done to accommodate layoffs. These steps were taken to minimize the operating cost and help to channel the revenue to the most needed aspects.

5.3.3 Employee Wellbeing Management

Since the emergence of Covid-19, the government has imposed many rules, work from home is one of them. To take care of the well-being and safety of their office employees, e-Hailing companies too have imposed work from home orders and some companies agreed to subsidize internet bills. Subsidy to purchase ergonomic chairs is also widely offered by employers. To protect the employees who have to come to the office every day, regular office area disinfection and common area such as pantry, meeting room disinfections were also carried on. These activities cost money to companies, however, many companies continue to do so to take off their employees.

5.3.4 Driver Partners and Delivery Partners Wellbeing Management

e-Hailing companies also turned their attention toward the driver-partners, delivery partners, and their passengers' safety and wellbeing. Many companies have taken responsibility for providing hand sanitizers and face masks to their driver-partners and delivery partners. A contactless delivery method was introduced for food delivery applications, where customers are encouraged to not receive the food by hand, instead to ask for the food to be placed somewhere at the delivery location. Later, the customer will collect the food from the mentioned place, without having to meet the delivery partners. A cashless payment method is also promoted to break the chain of Covid-19 and protect the delivery frontlines. Education and awareness of these methods were also promoted widely via the online platform. As a part of the driver partners' and delivery partners' wellbeing program, GrabTaxi has rolled out financial schemes where if any drivers or their family members have contracted Covid-19 and are hospitalized, Grab will give some financial compensation to the families. This has helped many driver-partners and delivery partners.

5.3.5 Carry out Corporate Social Responsibility Initiatives

Corporate Social Responsibility (CSR) is a philanthropic initiative taken by large companies as a part of giving back to the community. Usually, companies carry out volunteering works for the community or give charity to the needy. With the emergence of the Covid-19 pandemic, many families undergo a financial crisis. e-Hailing companies have contributed money to such families and donated cash to many homes and elderly care centers. This has also indirectly built a positive image towards the respective companies.

5.4 SUGGESTIONS FOR FUTURE PANDEMIC RECOVERY ACTION PLAN

In this section, the author gives suggestions on measures that can be taken by e-Hailing companies in combating a pandemic in the future.

Pre-Pandemic

There is a proverb that goes do not put all eggs in one basket. In the business world, it means companies should not focus on only one product and invest all their resources into it. Businesses must learn to diversify. Some combinations can sound ridiculous but they could eliminate the risk of losing all during an uncertain time, companies should pursue them. For example, when we hear the name Johnson & Johnson, only baby products and home health products come to our mind. However, Johnson & Johnson is also the maker of medical devices used in operation theatres. Therefore, even though their baby products get affected, they can continue to supply medical devices and vice versa.

Secondly, change is indeed the only constant thing in the world. Therefore, each business should have a business continuity plan to make sure the business sustains any hiccups. Things might go out of their hands, but walking into a crisis without a business continuity plan could be the worst choice ever.

Thirdly, poor self-hygiene is one of the main factors that contribute to the emergence and spread of any infectious diseases in the past. Therefore, to reduce the possibility of infection for future diseases, it is good to encourage all driver-partners and delivery partners to always sanitize their vehicles and wear a mask when feeling under the weather. Prevention is better than cure. Cleanliness and self-hygiene can avoid an outbreak.

During Pandemic

In an event of an outbreak of another global pandemic, always refer to the history to study how e-Hailing companies have survived during previous pandemics. The world has seen many global pandemics such as Ebola, Nipah Virus infection, Zika virus, and Influenza A H1N1. There are many lessons to learn from these histories.

Secondly, when it comes to headcount management, it is a good practice to implement pay-cut to the higher management team first, followed by the executive staff. This is to take care of the well-being of the employees and reduce unemployment among adults.

Thirdly, always ensure to provide proper customer service. It is vital to ensure no major complaints arise from customers and do not take any complaints lightly. Set up a team to investigate any complaints that flow in from customers, driver-partners, delivery partners, merchants, or third parties and take fair actions. Always abide by government rules. These practices are exceptionally important during pandemics because any negative images that are painted against the company will further hit the business. A lawsuit is the last thing that a company would want to face during a pandemic.

Post-Pandemic

A business to survive a pandemic itself would be a huge success. 2 scenarios can be drawn when discussing post-pandemic. Scenario one, the pandemic has completely ended and the world gets back to its original state before the pandemic. In this scenario, all businesses that survived the pandemic can get back to their initial strategy and slowly recover. For example, the marketing strategies being used before the pandemic can be identically re-used. On the other hand, scenario two depicts the declaration of endemic. When facing such a situation, proper business plans must be put in place on the assumption that the virus and its disease will continue to affect people and businesses. Innovation is extremely vital for scenario two. Businesses that do not innovate might face major challenges.

5.5 CONCLUSION

In the era of the Covid-19 pandemic, many economic sectors have been severely impacted. The e-Hailing industry too faced major impacts however, there were still many opportunities that arose with the shift of the market demand from ride services to food delivery and good delivery services. Unlike other industries such as the airline industry and tourism industry which were directly faced the consequences and had very little space to recover. Some companies even had to resort to mass retrenchment and bankruptcy. In the future, it is vital for all businesses regardless of nature should prepare a business continuity plan which includes threats from global health emergencies too.

ACKNOWLEDGEMENT

In completing this chapter, I am deeply indebted to my family who has supported me throughout this process. Not forgetting my love, Thomas Zavier for being strong support. Million thanks to Dr. Shathees Baskaran for giving me this opportunity and believing in me.

REFERENCES

Aldaihani, F. M. F., & Ali, N. A. (2018). Factors affecting customer loyalty in the restaurant service industry in Kuwait City, Kuwait. *Journal of International Business and Management*, *1*(2), 1-14.

Horsu E.N. & Yeboah S. T. (2015). Influence of Service Quality on Customer Satisfaction: A Study of Minicab Taxi Services in Cape Coast, Ghana. International Journal of Economics, Commerce, and Management. Vol. III, Issue 5 Pp. 1-14.

Hashim, J. H., Adman, M. A., Hashim, Z., Radi, M. F. M., & Kwan, S. C. (2021). COVID-19 epidemic in Malaysia: epidemic progression, challenges, and response. *Frontiers in public health, 9.*

Karim, W., Haque, A., Anis, Z., & Ulfy, M. A. (2020). The movement control order (MCO) for covid-19 crisis and its impact on tourism and hospitality sector in Malaysia. *International Tourism and Hospitality Journal, 3*(2), 1-7.

CHAPTER 6

SMEs: Vulnerability and Sustainability During Pandemic

Logaiswari Indiran & Santhi Ramanathan

6.1 INTRODUCTION

Small and medium-sized enterprises (SMEs) have been recognized as productive drivers comprising economic development and growth around the world, particularly in developing countries. They are deemed as one of the key contributors to the economy as a driver to reduce unemployment and contribute to the Gross Domestic Products (GDP). According to the World Bank Group (US), formal SMEs in developing countries contribute to 60 percent of the total employment, and 40 percent of the Gross National Product. SMEs occupy the largest portion of all business worldwide and contribute immensely through job creation, and provide high-quality goods and services.

SMEs are a remarkable driving factor in the world's economy. The importance of SMEs has also been recognized across countries by promoting entrepreneurship, simplifying the regulations and policy for SMEs, and providing various support to their development. Among the countries that provide high support to SMEs is Canada, where 98 percent of the total business establishments are from SMEs and they comprise one-third of the national GDP (Government of Canada, 2019). There are almost four million businesses in Mexico, based on Organisation for Economic Co-operation and Development (OECD) reports, and 99.8 percent are micro, small, and medium enterprises. In Mexico, Micro, Small & Medium Enterprises (MSMEs) account for 52 percent of the country's GDP and produce 72 percent of the country's official employment (OECD & IDEA Foundation, 2010). SMEs make up 99 percent of companies in Singapore, recruiting about 65 percent of its population and contributing to nearly half of the nominal GDP of the country in 2018.

In ASEAN, SMEs, such as the Philippines, play a decisive position in the development of the economy. They constitute

99.6 percent of all companies registered in the nation and employ 66.9 percent of the total labor force. Moreover, they account for 35 percent of the GDP of the world (Yeung, 2017). While in Indonesia, the most recent figure shows that 816,000 SMEs employ 7.9 million people which directly contributes 27 percent to the GDP. Besides contributing to the economy, SMEs also provide a huge impact on the socio-economy of an economy. Strong evidence is that MSMEs are the main pillar of socio-economic development in India. They provide 40 percent of India's workforce, 37.54 percent of GDP. 30 percent of total exports and contribute significantly to the GDP (SME Chamber of India, 2020). However, SMEs are facing a less desirable market climate in the UK, Germany, and France. Although tax policy is the key constraint in the first two economies, the lack of stability in the labour market and financial details on SMEs, as well as red tape, are the main constraints in France.

Like other countries, SMEs are the key drivers of economic development in Malaysia, where more than 90 percent of economic activities come from SMEs. In 2019, SMEs employed 66.2 percent of the employment in Malaysia, which impacted RM522.1 billion, or 38.9 percent, as major contributors to the GDP, which is one of the focal points in Malaysia (DOSM, 2019), SMEs in Malaysia are divided into three categories comprises micro, small, and medium-sized industries, defined based on sales turnover and the number of staff. SMEs are expected to continue to contribute to the overall national GDP by the end of the year 2030 by as much as 50 percent (Ministry of Entrepreneur Development, 2019). It is impossible to achieve that dream without support, a stimulus package, and continuing sustainable growth of SMEs. Therefore, the government will certify that the local SMEs remain robust and competitive in addressing economic challenges in any condition when they are vulnerable during the pandemic. This chapter will start with the dynamism of SMEs in Malaysia's economy, continued with the discussion on the vulnerability of SMEs during the Covid-19 pandemic, and provide the future direction toward sustainable practices in Malaysia.

6.2 DYNAMISMS OF SMEs IN THE MALAYSIAN ECONOMY

The primary drives of Small and medium-sized enterprises (SMEs) in Malaysia have been acknowledged widely, which mainly to promote economic development, increase job creation, foster innovation capability, and support sustainable development goals.

6.2.1 Economic Development

According to data released on 29 July 2020 by the Department of Statistics Malaysia (DOSM), the contribution of SMEs to total GDP rose to 38.9 percent in 2019, compared to 38.3 percent in 2018. In terms of production, at a constant 2015 rate, SME GDP stood at RM552.3 billion compared to RM1,421.5 billion for the overall value of total GDP. This represents a 5.8 percent rise in SME GDP in 2019, led by a solid 7.4 percent growth in the service sector. The growth momentum in the services sector was driven by the sub-sector of banking, insurance, real estate, and business services, which reported a higher 7.7 percent growth in 2019 (2018: 7.5 percent) as well as a steady expansion following company household spending in the F&B, retail trade, wholesale, and accommodation sub-sector. Since 2004, SMEs' growth has continued to outpace GDP.

6.2.2 Job Creation

In 2019, SMEs employed approximately 7.3 million workers, representing a rise of 3.0 percent from 2018, while adding 48.4 percent to state employment (2018: 48.0 percent). About 63.2 percent of total SME jobs, with the two highest primary sub-sectors; wholesale & retail trade, F&B, and accommodation. Manufacturing with 16.3 percent was also responsible for SME jobs, led by agriculture with 10.6 percent, construction with 9.7 percent, and mining & quarrying with 0.3 percent. The proportion of small and medium-sized enterprises employed was revised based on improvements in the methodology previously excluded by the government, the informal sector outside the agricultural sector, the non-registered enterprises in the agricultural sector, and the outsourcing of the total denominator computing activities for the estimation of SME jobs.

6.2.3 Foster Innovation Capability

The need and pressure for innovation capabilities are growing on businesses to prioritize competitive advantage to develop sustainability due to the increasing challenges of global competition, technology and knowledge-based economy, human resource advancement, and others. SMEs are also key players in the innovation ecosystem, as they contribute significantly to new product development, besides job and growth creation (De Marco et al., 2020; Storey, 2016). Therefore, after finding the market gap the technological advancement and disruption of the global supply chain drive the SMEs to reset and reshape new ideas and creativity to achieve sustainable business development (Lestari et al., 2018). SMEs sectors are heterogeneous, and these enable them to produce and diversify new products. They must also find the proper balance between interventions addressing novelty-related issues and more personalized solutions customized to the particular needs of the main categories of SMEs. The empirical study of 50 SMEs in the United Kingdom found that the innovation capabilities of SMEs were affected by the level of owner education, R&D focus, and increased human resources (Romijn & Albaladejo, 2000). Investment in creative activities continues to be on the increase among SMEs and leads to favourable outcomes for enterprises, irrespective of the source of investment funding (Piątkowski, 2020). Evidence also suggests that, as firm size decreases, the tendency to patent, which is a measure of the development of new technical information, appears to increase. Innovation and technologies policies that stimulate innovation development in SMEs. Aligned with the same initiative, Malaysia has embarked on various projects, innovation activities, and R&D expenditures for Bumiputera entrepreneurs. The Government of Malaysia has set up various agencies for Bumiputera SME programs offered primarily Perbadanan Nasional Berhad (PNS), Majlis Amanah Rakyat (MARA), Perbadanan Usahawan Nasional Berhad (PUNB), Tabung Ekonomi Kumpulan Usaha Niaga (TEKUN), Amanah Ikhtiar Malaysia (AIM) and CEDAR. Skillful and creative Bumiputera entrepreneurs are the primary target of these initiatives. Research shows that technology and innovation approaches are a channel for businesses to penetrate and nurture overseas markets (Amankwah-Amoah Osabutey and Egbetokun, 2018).

6.3 VULNERABILITY OF SMEs AND BATTLES AGAINST COVID-19

Various publications and reports both at the international and national levels have covered a wide range of analyses and findings of Covid-19 and its impact on various economic activities. According to the World Economic Outlook Update,

June 2020, global economic growth has been depicted as moving downward with a growth rate projected at −4.9 percent. It's not a strange occurrence to have a downward trend indicator during the crisis, but the pandemic has brought serious lockdown. Although the lockdown or movement restrictions have helped to slow down or stopped the spread of the virus and save lives, on the other hand, it sparked the worst economic crisis since World War II (The World Bank, 2020). In the worst case of the second wave of this pandemic, OECD's June 2020 Economic Outlook has projected a 7.6 percent fall by the end of 2020, followed by a moderate recovery of 2.8 percent in 2021 (OECD, 2020). With these tragic figures, the impact of Covid-19 on unemployment worldwide is expected to increase from 5.3 million to 24.7 million, indicating the potential challenges and hurdles for companies, particularly for those small and medium-sized enterprises (ILO, 2020).

Small and medium-sized enterprises (SMEs) have often been more affected and more vulnerable than large firms (OECD, 2020). According to the compilation of surveys produced by OCDC (2020), about 42 surveys in 20 countries across the globe from 10th February 2020 to 20th June 2020, were conducted to discover the impact of Covid-19 on SMEs. This in a way shows the increasing concerns among SMEs. Malaysia is certainly not exceptional in this context.

According to the survey conducted by the SME Association of Malaysia among 1,713 members, the Covid-19 pandemic has caused a higher risk of closure for about one-quarter of Malaysia's small and medium-sized enterprises over the second half of the year. The survey revealed the critical situation of 22 percent of the respondents having sufficient cash flow for them to survive for a month, about 27 percent and 31 percent to sustain till November and December respectively (The Edge Markets, 2020). Besides the financial difficulties which include cash flow-related issues, bankruptcy, and reaching the appropriate stimulus packages, SMEs are also found to be affected by problems related to operation and supply chain disruption as well as difficulties in predicting the future path of business (Omar et al., 2020). Along with these problems, Azmi et al. (2020) conducted a survey on 348 SMEs in Malaysia and discovered the duties and responsibilities of staff, administrative skill and knowledge, and financial credibility as SMEs battle throughout this pandemic.

6.3.1 Most Vulnerable Sectors

Among the most vulnerable sectors during the current pandemic and crisis are transportation, construction, retail cum wholesale trading, aviation, hotels or lodging, food and beverages, real estate, professional and personal services, such as hairdressing (OECD, 2020) as well as businesses related to arts, education, entertainment, and recreation (International Monetary Fund, 2020).

However, several key characteristics would determine the vulnerability of SMEs during pandemics or crises. Firstly, whether the SMEs are more labour-intensive, thus affected by employees' being locked down, or whether they are adequately flexible to modify their business model when necessary (Yi, 2020). Secondly, SMEs' limitations in terms of financial resources, in the form of liquidity or assets, are considered a common factor that often pushes them towards shutdown or exit the market. Thirdly, the innovation capabilities (Kashif et al., 2020) of SMEs, may help them to adopt alternative business models, integrate technology or ICT (Tong and Gong, 2020), and develop networking or partnerships to enhance or sustain the business operations during the crisis.

6.3.2 Financial Risk

Financial issues are always being the most fundamental factor that determines SMEs' well-being. Theedgemarkets. com (2020) highlighted some key points on the financial capabilities of SMEs as a result of an online survey conducted among 15,627 SMEs in Malaysia. The result indicated that most SMEs are in a very tight condition in terms of cash flow particularly and the condition is expected to aggravate even after Movement Control Order (MCO), with the reasons of various commitments comprising worker's salary, rent, and other statutory expenditures. Department of Statistics Malaysia (2020) and Yi (2020) highlighted a similar pattern of growth faced by several larger enterprises and micro-sized enterprises, they may not be able to survive for more than two months and even in some cases end up surviving for shorter periods due to lack of cash. Another research conducted by Omar et al. (2020) on a small group of SMEs has revealed the survival strategies implemented by those SMEs during this pandemic and under the MCO situation. The internal ability to adopt the financial and marketing survival strategies during a pandemic varies depending on the type of business activities and the assets or resources retained. The findings precisely indicated that during the pandemic or crisis phase, an accumulated financial resource of the organization is a very effective instrument for business continuity, while other assets and skills enable businesses to adapt to new business opportunities.

Based on the current circumstances faced by SMEs, the Malaysian government has launched and executed various financing assistance and facilities. PRIHATIN Economic Stimulus Package 2020 with allocation amounted to RM3.3 billion and followed by the Additional PRIHATIN SME Economic Stimulus Package (PRIHATIN SME+) with an additional allocation of RM10 billion was launched to support SMEs in overcoming the uncertainty of business administration and operations (Bank Negara Malaysia, 2020). Among the schemes or programs established to assist SMEs during this difficult period are Special Relief Facility (SRF), All Economic Sectors (AES) Facility, Agrofood Facility (AF), SME Automation and Digitalisation Facility (ADF), Targeted Relief and Recovery Facility (TRRF), High Tech Facility – National Investment Aspirations (HTF-NIA), and Micro Enterprises Facility (MEF). SMEs are also given financing assistance via Credit Guarantee Corporation Malaysia Berhad's (CGC) BizMula-i and BizWanita-i schemes. The business financing referral platform consists of banks (commercial and Islamic) and development financial institutions controlled by BNM also made available for SMEs for the financing facilities. In line with these offers, the Ministry of Entrepreneur Development and Cooperatives (MEDAC), through its agencies such as Tekun Nasional, SME Bank, SME Corp, and Bank Rakyat, has disbursed some RM47.4 billion in financing to 485,000 micro and SME entrepreneurs as well as cooperatives as of July 2020 (SMEcorp, 2020). In the context of particular sector-based stimulus measures, the government opened the tourism fund to support SMEs in the tourism sector to remain sustainable (OECD, 2020).

6.3.3 Digital Divide

According to the World Bank Group (2018), the state of digitalization by Malaysian businesses remains below the global average level. It has been reported that SMEs perform quite poorly in digitalization and thus it is evident the existence of a digital divide among businesses in Malaysia (World Bank Group, 2018). This state of SMEs' engagement towards digitalization seems to be the root cause of the struggles faced by SMEs to sustain during the current pandemic and MCO.

The inability of SMEs in switching their business operation to the digital platform during the movement control order had led to inefficiency and business slowdown.

A study of Workday Digital Agility Index published a survey done in the Asia Pacific covering the field of human resources, finance, and Information Technology and the response of business leaders and executives towards digital transformation. The study found that about 25 percent of Malaysian companies have expedited their digital transformation strategies as a result of the lockdown or movement control order implemented due to the Covid-19 pandemic, while 60 percent have slowed down (Business Today, 2020). In addition to this trend, within one week of the movement control order (MCO), closed to 69 percent of SMEs have experienced a more than 50 percent drop in business and subsequently discovered the concern among SMEs on the importance of learning new skills including digital skills at this point of time (Malay Mail, 2020). Despite this scenario, the Malaysia Digital Economy Corporation (MDEC) expected a growth of 20 percent in e-commerce's contribution to the digital economy in 2020 which could be due to the overwhelming performance of online shopping (Yi, 2020). Being aware of SMEs' struggles connecting towards digitalization is partly due to financial constraints, MDEC via the short-term economic recovery plan Penjana has apportioned RM700 million to support SMEs in adopting digitalization (The Sunday Daily, 2020). Besides financial issues being a challenge for SMEs to digitize their businesses, they also experienced difficulties in terms of infrastructure capabilities such as online connectivity with customers, suppliers as well as employees under work-from-home (WFH) arrangement (Ernst & Young, 2020). The Covid-19 pandemic has made the SMEs in Malaysia move progressively toward digitalization to remain sustainable in the long term (BERNAMA, 2020).

6.3.4 Changed Customer Behaviours

Covid-19 pandemic and the lockdown have impacted a huge reduction in consumption growth for most economies, which eventually had led to huge disruption to domestic activity (IMF, 2020). Businesses, including SMEs, face a decline in global demand for their goods and services (OECD, 2020). A drastic change in customers' preference and demand due to the pandemic and MCO had steered great impact on SMEs' production revenue and their ability to sustain in the marketplace. This change in customer behaviors includes the change in types of goods and services between essential and non-essential, quantity of goods and services, timing of their purchases, and finally change in preference towards online versus face-to-face purchasing. This variation in customers' behavior could be due to the concern of social distancing or fear of infections, customers' conditions such as loss of job, income, and savings, all in, weaken consumer confidence and aggravated the reduction of spending and consumption (IMF, 2020). This condition seems to be disastrous for SMEs in sectors such as tourism, hotels and accommodation sector, transportation

Marketing Insight (2020) surveyed people's perceived impacts of movement control order in Kuala Lumpur and Penang. The survey indicated that the changes in consumers' buying behaviour throughout movement control order are being one of the reasons for SMEs to transform their business operation into a digital platform. This concludes that the understanding of SMEs' survival strategies is being a very important factor for businesses to sustain during this difficult time.

6.4 FUTURE DIRECTION TOWARDS SUSTAINABLE PRACTICES

Several reviews, research, and surveys on sustainability, sustainable growth of Small and medium-sized enterprises (SMEs), and Sustainable Manufacturing Practices (SMP) from the Malaysian perspective reveal that there is lacking in terms of attention, strategies, and plans or implementation that would assist the practitioners and policymakers towards achieving sustainable growth of SMEs (Yusoff et al., 2018; Norsiah Hami et al., 2018; Lee, 2017). Subsequently, this research initiates had proposed an integrated framework comprising the factors within the domain of SMEs, internal intangible factors portrayed as having a significant effect on the dimensions of economic perspective of sustainable growth (Yusoff et al., 2018). In line with this, the government perceived that Malaysia's SMEs should start thinking about sustainability or embracing sustainable practices to penetrate new export markets, as more established markets already have certain principles in place. Malaysia External Trade and Development Corp (Matrade) and the Ministry of International Trade and Industry (MITI) together aimed to create more consciousness towards sustainability among Malaysian SMEs (The Edge Financial Daily, 2019). A recent study on the effect of organizational culture on the sustainable growth of SMEs reveals that maintaining or installing innovative organizational culture by manufacturing SMEs would have a positive and significant effect on enhancing efficient sustainable growth (Nimfa et al., 2020).

In addressing the current and post era of the Covid-19 pandemic, ecological disruption, climate destabilization, and other threats demand great leadership and sustainable efforts (theedgemarkets.com, 2020). Thus, during the current and post-COVID periods, SMEs are expected to move beyond their current agility and continue to increase their value proposition to remain important and sustained. Innovation, digitalization, and collaborating or networking would be the key factors for entrepreneurs as well as a fundamental characteristic of its business model in the post-pandemic era (BERNAMA, 2020).

6.4.1 Sustainable Development Policies

The support of the government or public sector plays a vital role in the success and sustainability of SMEs (Kashif et al., 2020) and is particularly essential to ensure a smooth recovery of the economy. International Monetary Fund (2020) study highlights the importance of proper targeting of fiscal interventions to support SMEs which would significantly reduce the rate of business failures at significant fiscal costs (IMF, 2020). In the case of South Korea, the government offered an income tax reduction of 80 percent to credit and debit card users to stimulate pre-payment and pre-purchasing and the government of Germany reduced the VAT by three points until the end of 2020 (OECD, 2020). In Malaysia, the government helping SMEs through its key initiative, called PENJANA spending about RM70 million as part of the economic stimulus package (BERNAMA, 2020).

Besides safeguarding the cash flows of SMEs to ensure their sustainability as the SMEs' importance increases, the concern on the wastage of inputs or underutilized capacity (Lee et al., 2017) and their threats to the environment is being another concern (NST, 2020). As such, developing strategies to reduce wastage and being mindful of the potential environmental degradation, are both equally important for SMEs in achieving sustainability. The case of Sungai Selangor pollution and resulting unplanned water damage that affected almost 1.2 million households was not the first incident of its kind. SMEs are expected to attain their goals without restraining the ability of future generations to meet their needs and wants.

Dr. Devika Nadarajah in her article entitled SMEs can play their part in creating a sustainable future (NSTP, 2020), stressed the need for traditional business practitioners to shift their business model towards environmentally cum sustainability-oriented practices. Among those are the need to emphasize dealing assets or resources efficiently to yield goods and services at ideal value without leading to waste; monitor and modify SMEs' energy consumption mechanisms towards renewable resources; SME Corp to collaborate with relevant government authorities to provide environmental related training and awareness; policy interferences through tax deductions; creating and providing viable opportunities for SMEs to nurture green business models across various industries or sectors. Besides this well-designed proposal, Yi (2020) has written a policy brief based on findings from a webinar, SMEs Beyond the MCO – Lessons from the PRIHATIN Stimulus, participated by speakers representing the Malaysian Retail Chain Association (MRCA), The Association of Bumiputera Women in Business and Profession (PENIAGAWATI), SME Corporation Malaysia, Small and Medium Enterprises Association Malaysia (SAMENTA) and Malaysian International Chamber of Commerce and Industry (MICCI) respectively. This policy brief has compiled opinions from the SMEs and generated valuable feedback for the construction of an appropriate public policy. Among the most crucial recommendations are the need to formalize the SMEs that operate as part of the informal sector to conduct their businesses appropriately and so that would be eligible for the benefits of social protection; to let SMEs participate in the procurement process, and review internal measures and rules to facilitate digital adoption.

6.4.2 Sustainable Digital Infrastructure

OECD (2020) report contained a segment of critical review on nine different surveys discovering the SMEs' capabilities and new business practices which include teleworking and digitalization. Among the 3 major trends that can be identified from the review is the attitude of SMEs shifting toward digitalization, an increase in the perceived importance of digitalization towards firms' flexibility and responsiveness, and lastly, the existence of a gap in the pervasiveness of digitalization due to insufficient of infrastructure and employee's skills to use digital tools. SMEs and digitalization had become interconnected dimensions that were required for the resilience of SMEs during this COVID-19 pandemic and economic uncertainty. The government's support for SMEs to digitize their businesses mainly focuses on increasing the digital skills of entrepreneurs, business owners, and their employees, and secondly is to expanding the access to digital infrastructure, tools, and techniques (OECD, 2020).

Despite financial turbulences among SMEs brought by the Covid-19 pandemic, the adoption and investment in new technologies to enhance operational efficiency and embrace a massive benefit towards sustainability has become an ultimate direction for many SMEs (BERNAMA, 2020; Yi, 2020). A study conducted by the University Consortium of Malaysia found that the use of digital technology would increase the efficiency and productivity of SMEs significantly. SMEs using social media experienced a productivity increase of 26 percent, while those participating in e-commerce experienced a productivity increase of 27 percent (Tong and Gong, 2020). Realizing the importance of climbing on this digitalization bandwagon at this critical juncture, SMEs must be exposed to and equipped with a complete set of information on the government's offers, schemes, programs, and incentives to make viable choices or decisions and move towards sustainable growth.

In Malaysia, the government proposes seven main digitalization capacities to be incorporated by small and medium-sized enterprises. The capacities fall into various key areas such as digital marketing and sales, Electronic point of sales (e-POS) system, HR payroll system or CRM, procurement, E-commerce, remote working, EPF, accounting as well as tax (MDEC, 2020).

6.4.3 Digital Literacy

During this Covid-19 critical period, continued research is being conducted on the adaptability or agility of SMEs towards digital applications or solutions. The findings from those research seem to be consistent in terms of strongly highlighting the positive correlation between digitalization and cost efficiency as well as the sustainability of SMEs. Besides the digital infrastructure, digital literacy as another dimension of the digitalization platform is also being a major concern in the context of Malaysian SMEs' survival, during the pre-Covid19 pandemic (World Bank Group, 2018) as well as throughout the pandemic and MCOs.

Digital literacy is not a recent concept or trending formation and was referred to as computer literacy during the 1980s. According to Buckingham (2015), digital or computer literacy appears to quantify a marginal set of skills that will facilitate u the changes in consumer's buying behaviour throughout movement control in order ser to operate the computer software resources and tools as well as to search for basic information effectively. However, the recent era of digitalization, particularly the digitalization of the production-based industries is driven by various technologies advancement and convergence such as Additive Manufacturing, Artificial Intelligence, Big Data Analytics, Advance materials such as nano-structures, cybersecurity, Simulation, Cloud Computing, Augmented Reality, Internet of Things (IoT), Autonomous Robots and System Integration (MITI, 2018). In June 2018, SME Corp. Malaysia and Huawei Technologies Malaysia commissioned a study to explore the state of Information and Communications Technology (ICT) adoption among 2,033 small and medium-sized enterprises in the services, manufacturing, construction, and agriculture sectors and representing all regions. The survey revealed that SMEs are not well-versed in using digital technologies for three aspects, namely, connecting to more customers, computerizing business operations, and in terms of data protection. SMEs are also found to be lacking in terms of knowledge and awareness of usage and benefits of social media marketing and e-commerce including cloud, IoT, and data analytics.

The gap between technological advancement and SMEs' agility has to be consistently scrutinized and assessed based on a standard benchmarking index or system. It's a clear indication that the definition of digitalization of SMEs is no longer limited to operating the computer system and processes, but has extended to greater scope which required SMEs to remodel the business practices based on ICT, which includes administration, operations, sales, and marketing (Huawei Technologies & SME Corp, 2018). Thus, digital literacy would play a vital role in driving Malaysia, particularly SMEs toward sustainable digital practice. Following this proposition, besides accelerating the awareness of the benefits of digitalizing, training and upskilling are essential in enhancing digital literacy which may eventually improve the SMEs' technical knowledge and competencies.

6.4.4 Connectional Intelligence

The Covid-19 pandemic led to a long-lasting impact on local as well as global value chains. In this scenario, the connection and networking elements have a proactive function in sustaining the business operations among SMEs during MCOs or lockdowns. SMEs usually have inadequate suppliers, limited connections, and networks which compresses their flexibility and agility to opt for alternative ways of logistics and transportation (OECD, 2020). OECD highlighted two potential avenues for public action in strengthening the connections and networks among SMEs. First, the government may provide companies with timely market information and intelligence that can help SMEs build extensive networks as well as diversify their supplier base. The second is by supporting SMEs in identifying, evaluating, and managing risks by sharing information on supply chains.

In Malaysia, as part of the government's PENJANA initiative, the cooperation between large corporations or companies with the government would be certainly an essential factor in an attempt to kick-start the economy, in a way to help SMEs succeed in this "new normal". The government's role in nurturing resilience by implementing public-private partnerships would be a great deal in empowering the local SMEs (BERNAMA, 2020). Partnership with the international community is also curial for SMEs, particularly for export-focused companies, as the contribution to Malaysia's exports in 2018 is only 18 percent. This has urged MATRADE's commitment to continuously work with other ministries and agencies to further develop SMEs' export capabilities across all sectors (The Edge Financial Daily, 2019). In addition, to recover and expand the export market or internationalization activities involving SMEs, the healthcare system, existing trade, and investment policies need to be strengthened, particularly, the connectional or network intelligence or capabilities among SMEs which may safeguard their sustainability.

6.5 CONCLUSION

According to IMF (2020), overall, the fiscal deficits and debt level are expected to increase dramatically at the end of 2021 and the governments are expected to retain their current structure over the forecast periods until the end of 2021. Generally, for both advanced and emerging market economies, financial conditions are expected to remain approximately at current levels. In Malaysia, the government is optimizing the resources available to execute those initiatives announced and being implemented, with the expectation that SMEs would be able to gain the benefits and sustain themselves in the marketplace. The impact of the Covid-19 pandemic on the Malaysian economy, particularly on SMEs can be regarded as an unprecedented phenomenon. The current challenges faced by SMEs would be a great lesson for all stakeholders to embrace more sustainable business practices which focus on long-term commitments with progressive policies toward SMEs' sustainability.

REFERENCES

Abd Elkhalek, A. M. A. (2019). SMEs' Contribution to Sustainable Development; an Applied Study Focusing on OECD Countries.

Amos Tong and Rachel Gong (2020). Digitalisation of firms: Challenges in the digital economy, VIEWS 42/20, Khazanah Research Institute

Azmi, W., Aida, I., & Diana, A.W. (2020). The role of strategic management in growth of small and medium enterprises (SMEs) in Malaysia. e-Bangi Journal of Social Sciences and Humanities, 17(1), 108-124.

BERNAMA (2020). Helping small businesses navigate through COVID-19 recovery by Leo Chow Chief Executive Officer of Lazada Malaysia. Retrieved from https://www.bernama.com/en/thoughts/news.php?id=1860516

Buckingham, D. (2015). Defining digital literacy: What do young people need to know about digital media? Medienbildung in Neuen Kulturräumen Die Deutschprachige Und Britische Diskussion. 2015. 21-34. Retrieved from https://www.researchgate.net/publication/284919482_Defining_digital_literacy_What_do_young_people_need_to_know_about_digital_media

Business Today (2020). Workday finds only 25 percent of Malaysian organisations have accelerated digital transformation plans. Retrieved from Workday finds only 25 percent of Malaysian organisations have accelerated digital transformation plans | Business Today

De Marco, C. E., Martelli, I., & Di Minin, A. (2020). European SMEs' engagement in open innovation When the important thing is to win and not just to participate, what should innovation policy do?. Technological Forecasting and Social Change, 152, 119843.

Department of Statistics Malaysia (2020). Main Findings of Special Survey 'Effects of COVID-19 on the Economy and Companies/Business Firms'- Round. DOSM, Malaysia. Retrieved from Department of Statistics Malaysia Official Portal (dosm.gov.my)

Department of Statistics Malaysia. (2020). Report of Special Survey on Effects of Covid-19 on Economy and Individual (Round 1). Retrieved from https://www.dosm.gov.my/.

Donbesuur, F., Ampong, G. O. A., Owusu-Yirenkyi, D., & Chu, I. (2020). Technological innovation, organizational innovation and international performance of SMEs: The moderating role of domestic institutional environment. Technological Forecasting and Social Change, 161, 120252.

Ernst & Young. (2020). COVID-19: Impact on Malaysian business. Retrieved September 9, 2020, from https://www.ey.com/en_my/take-5-business-alert/ covid-19-impact-on-malaysian-businesses

Government of Canada (2019). Key small business statistics. Government of Canada. Retrieved July 12, 2018, from https://www.ic.gc.ca/eic/site/061.nsf/eng/h_03090.html.

Hadi, S., & Supardi, S. (2020). Revitalization Strategy for Small and Medium Enterprises after Corona Virus Disease Pandemic (Covid-19) in Yogyakarta. J. Xian Univ. Archit. Technol, 12, 4068-4076.

Hamburg, I. (2020). Facilitating Lifelong Learning in SMEs Towards SDG4. Advances in Social Sciences Research Journal, 7(9).

Hanifah, H., Halim, H. A., Ahmad, N. H., & Vafaei-Zadeh, A. (2019). Emanating the key factors of innovation performance: leveraging on the innovation culture among SMEs in Malaysia. Journal of Asia Business Studies.

Huawei Technologies & SME Corp (2018). Accelerating Malaysian Digital SMEs: Escaping the Computerization Trap. Retrieved from https://www.huawei.com/minisite/ accelerating-malaysia-digital-smes/index.html

Huynh, T. (2020). A study on the effect of transformational leadership on work motivation: A case of employees at small and medium enterprises in Vietnam. Management Science Letters, 11(1), 41-48.

International Labour Organization. (2020). COVID-19 and the world of work: Impact and policy responses, ILO Monitor 1st Edition. Retrieved from https://www.ilo.org/global/about-the-ilo/WCMS_738753/lang--en/index.htm

Kashif, M., Asif, M. U., Ali, A., Asad, M., Asad, M., Chethiyar, S. D. M. & Vedamanikam, M. (2020). Managing and Implementing Change Successfully with Respect to COVID-19: A Way Forward for SMEs. PEOPLE: International Journal of Social Sciences, 6(2), 609-624.

Lee, M. D., Djubair, R. A., & Ngu, H. J. (2017). Sustainability Paradigm for Malaysian Manufacturing SMEs: An Operations Research Approach. International Journal of Business and Technopreneurship, 7(3), 355-368.

MalayMail (2020). Covid-19: After MCO, survey finds nearly 70pc SMEs lost half income. Retrieved from Covid-19: After MCO, survey finds nearly 70pc SMEs lost half income | Malaysia | Malay Mail

Marketing Insight. (2020). Sentiment study on the impact of Covid 19 MCO on Malaysians. Retrieved from https://marketingmagazine.com.my/.

MDEC (2020). Propelling SMEs into the Digital World. Retrieved from https://mdec.my/digital-economy-initiatives/for-the-industry/sme-digitalisation-grant/

Ministry Of International Trade And Industry (2018). Industry 4WRD: National Policy on Industry 4.0. Ministry of International Trade & Industry (MITI). Retrieved from https://www.miti.gov.my/miti/resources/ National percent20Policy percent20on percent20Industry percent204.0/Industry4WRD_Final.pdf

Muhyiddin, M.Y. (2020). Additional PRIHATIN SME Economic Stmulus Package (PRIHATIN SME+), Speech Text – Prime Minister Department. Retrieved from https://pmo.gov.my/2020/04.

Nimfa, D. T., Latiff, A. S. A., Wahab, S. A., & Raj, P. E. Effect of Organisational Culture On Sustainable Growth Of SMEs: Mediating Role of Innovation Competitive Advantage.

Norsiah Hami, Fadhilah Mat Yamin, Shafini Mohd Shafie, Mohd Razali Muhamad, Zuhriah Ebrahim (2018). Sustainable Manufacturing Practices Among SMEs in Malaysia. International Journal of Technology (2018) 8: 1658-1667.

NSTP (2020). SMEs can play their part in creating a sustainable future. Retrieved from https://www.nst.com.my/opinion/columnists/2020/09/626504/smes-can-play-their-part-creating-sustainable-future

OECD y "Fundación IDEA" (2010) Consolidación de la competencia económica y la mejora regulatoria para la competitividad en México, Estudio de caso. Puebla, Prácticas y políticas exitosas para la mejora regulatoria y el emprendedurismo a nivel subnacional. México.

OECD, "Coronavirus (COVID-19): SME Policy Responses," Note, OECD July 2020. Retrieved from https://www.oecd.org/coronavirus/policy-responses/coronavirus-covid-19-sme-policy-responses-04440101/#section-d1e18435

OECD (2020). Coronavirus (COVID-19): SME policy responses. Retrieved from https://www.oecd.org/coronavirus/policy-responses/coronavirus-covid-19-sme-policy-responses-04440101/#section-d1e18435

OECD (2020). Economic Outlook June 2020. Retrieved from http://www.oecd.org/economic-outlook/june-2020/

OECD. (2020). New OECD outlook on the global economy. Retrieved from https://www.oecd.org/coronavirus.

OECD (2020), "The impact of COVID-19 on SME financing: A special edition of the OECD Financing SMEs and Entrepreneurs Scoreboard", OECD SME and Entrepreneurship Papers, No. 22, OECD Publishing, Paris. Available at https://doi.org/10.1787/ecd81a65-en.

Omar, A. R. C., Ishak, S., & Jusoh, M. A. (2020). The impact of Covid-19 Movement Control Order on SMEs' businesses and survival strategies. Geografia-Malaysian Journal of Society and Space, 16(2).

Piątkowski, M. J. (2020). Results of SME Investment Activities: A Comparative Analysis among Enterprises Using and Not Using EU Subsidies in Poland. Administrative Sciences, 10(1), 4.

Poon, W. C., Mohamad, O., & Yusoff, W. F. W. (2020). Examining the antecedents of ambidextrous behaviours in promoting creativity among SMEs in Malaysia. Global Business Review, 21(3), 645-662.

Prime Minister's Office of Malaysia. (2020). Prihatin Rakyat Economic Stimulus Package (PRIHATIN) Speech Text - Speech by YAB Tan Sri Dato' Haji Muhyiddin Bin Haji Mohd Yassin Perdana Menteri Malaysia. Retrieved from https://www.pmo.gov.my/2020.

SMEcorp (2020). MEDAC says will continue to give attention to SMEs post-COVID-19. Retrieved from https://www.smecorp.gov.my/index.php/en/resources/2015-12-21-10-55-22/news/4204-medac-says-will-continue-to-give-attention-to-smes-post-covid-19

Storey, D. J. (2016). Understanding the small business sector. Routledge.

Theedgemarkets.com. (2020). 25 percent of SMEs face closure risk amid new wave of Covid-19. Retrieved from https://www.theedgemarkets.com/article/25-smes-face-closure-risk-amid-new-wave-covid19

Theedgemarkets.com. (2020). Malaysia March manufacturing output dented by Covid-19 pandemic. Retrieved from https://www.theedgemarkets.com/article/malaysia-march-manufacturing-output-dented-covid19-pandemic

Theedgemarkets.com. (2020). Take a leaf from Nestlé Malaysia's green leadership. Retrieved from https://www.theedgemarkets.com/content/advertise/take-a-leaf-from-nestle-malaysia-green-leadership

The Edge Financial Daily. (2019). Start thinking about sustainable business practices, SMEs told. Retrieved from https://www.theedgemarkets.com/article/start-thinking-about-sustainable-business-practices-smes-told

The New Straits Times. (2020). Covid-19: Movement Control Order imposed with only essential sectors operating. Retrieved from https://www.nst.com.my/news/nation/2020/03/575177/covid-19-movement-control-order-imposed-only-essential-sectors-operating

The New Straits Times. (2020). SMEs can play their part in creating a sustainable future. Retrieved from https://www.nst.com.my/opinion/columnists/2020/09/626504/smes-can-play-their-part-creating-sustainable-futuree

The Star Online. (2020). Special online survey to study effects of Covid-19 on Malaysians, economy. Retrieved from https://www.thestar.com.my/news/nation/2020/03/23.

Voon Zhen Yi (2020). Struggle of Malaysian SMEs During the COVID-19 Pandemic, POLICY BRIEF May 2020, KSI Strategic Institute for Asia Pacific.

The Sunday Daily (2020). MDEC: E-commerce expected to grow 20 percent this year despite MCO. Retrieved from MDEC: E-commerce expected to grow 20 percent this year despite MCO (thesundaily.my)

The World Bank (2020). COVID-19 to Plunge Global Economy into Worst Recession since World War II, Press Release June 8, Washington. Retrieved from https://www.worldbank.org/en/news/press-release/2020/06/08/covid-19-to-plunge-global-economy-into-worst-recession-since-world-war-ii

Wasiuzzaman, S., Nurdin, N., Abdullah, A. H., & Vinayan, G. (2020). Creditworthiness and access to finance of SMEs in

Malaysia: do linkages with large firms matter?. Journal of Small Business and Enterprise Development.

Westman, L., Moores, E., & Burch, S. L. Bridging the governance divide: The role of SMEs in urban sustainability interventions. Cities, 108, 102944.

Yeung, H. W. C. (2017). Global production networks and foreign direct investment by small and medium enterprises in ASEAN. Transnational corporations, 24(2), 1-42.

Yi, V. Z. (2020). Struggle of Malaysian SMEs During the COVID-19 Pandemic.

Yusoff, T., Wahab, S. A., Latiff, A. S., Osman, S. I., Zawawi, N. F., & Fazal, S. A. (2018). Sustainable Growth in SMEs: A Review from the Malaysian Perspective. J. Mgmt. & Sustainability, 8, 43.

CHAPTER 7

COVID Business Matrix for a Remade World

Shathees Baskaran

7.1 INTRODUCTION

Despite the fact that there is no established strategy for coping with a catastrophe of the size of COVID-19, organizations are required to be always ready to manage the risks as they come. However, organizations do not simply manage risk.

They exploit the risk as a source of growth since it allows them to engage in a forward-thinking orientation to achieve what it wants to do, swiftly and safely. Given the pandemic's magnitude and complexity, there's a good chance that the COVID-19 recovery phase will need unprecedented levels of coordination, communication, and reconfiguration of current business models. As traditional organizations crumbled, disruption reigned supreme. Businesses all across the world had to respond quickly and decisively to the pandemic's problems. Despite multiple predictions about the future of businesses and organizations, one will need to acknowledge that the businesses will reopen and resume eventually. As the businesses recover, it's critical for the organizations to react to the future competitive landscape, determining which changes brought on by the crisis will serve as the "new normal." As organizations enter the next phase of the recovery, now is the time for these organizations to look for and grasp the possibilities that are developing by building strategic resilience for future sustainability. In view of this, the chapter introduces a COVID Business Matrix (known as CoBuM), discussing four characteristics namely Products and Services, channels, Infrastructure, and Skills in designing post-COVID-19, new normal business strategies in response to COVID-19 challenges. Organizations that take appropriate actions by reconfiguring their present business models now will be better positioned to take advantage of the possibilities that will emerge as the post-COVID-19 recovery unfolds which would allow these organizations to continue to succeed in their marketplaces.

7.2 ORGANIZATIONAL FLEXIBILITY

The business world is very unpredictable, complicated, and chaotic nowadays. These changes are rising at a quicker rate making a business environment extremely dynamic forcing organizations to work harder to sustain in hyper turbulent conditions. As a result, understanding the constantly changing environment in which companies operate has become increasingly relevant and crucial. Hence, organizations that can adapt properly to shifting degrees of environmental uncertainty, according to the structural contingency hypothesis, will be more effective. One of the most important aspects of success in a timed competition is flexibility. The idea behind this notion is to be able to adjust organizational procedures to follow suit the changes in the internal and external environment. In a nutshell, the ability of an organization to react to a changing environment is referred to as flexibility which pertains to various abilities of an organization. Flexibility is required at both the strategic and operational levels to achieve the organization's impact.

In an ideal situation, practically all management approaches should be built on an openness to the environment and a quick response to changing circumstances. A flexible organization is well prepared to engage in continuous opportunities exploration in good as well as bad times. The organization is well-positioned to maneuver its course by adapting itself to the present business conditions to succeed commercially. Flexibility in the organization is exhibited only when the organization could strike a balance between exploration of opportunities and deployment of assets according to the need of present business conditions. When meeting and achieving the organizational expectation is difficult and strategic surprise is imminent, organizational flexibility is viewed as an important strategic alternative in turbulent business environments.

The key principles that determine organizational flexibility need continuous attention. The research has witnessed multiple views, arguments, consensus as well as debates in explaining the organizational flexibility phenomenon. Nevertheless, the objective approach that can be used to explain organizational flexibility is evolving continuously. Therefore, it is important to acknowledge that the measurement of organizational flexibility is a complicated issue that needs continuous exploration to change the principles that set the flexible framework for the organizations to follow and implement.

Despite various approaches introduced in the past, this chapter introduces a new matrix that can be used to explain organizational flexibility. This matrix is known as COVID Business Matrix. Due to its evolving nature, there is no common framework to explain organizational flexibility. This shortcoming can be attributed to the changing nature of the organization and its controllable and uncontrollable operating environment. In this vein, the COVID Business Matrix is attempted to address five fundamental principles that allow organizations to build their resilience and agility to remain sustainable in pressing business conditions.

7.3 THE COVID BUSINESS MATRIX

Organizations are now taking a more holistic and strategic approach, including all aspects of sustainability, and developing their future business models and corresponding business strategies by also relying on partnerships for assistance as necessary. In doing so, organizations' decisions are required to be cogent, indicating the quality of being clear, logical, and convincing and also strong decision-making that has true premises in providing conclusive support for the organizations' to plan its way forward.

The author premised that cogency in the organization is not a standalone process. Instead, it is driven by four other important pillars which allow the organization to remain cogent at different times of business growth as well as disruptions. Accordingly, the four pillars identified were Objectivity, Versatility, Immunity, and as well as Diversity with Cogency being at the center of these pillars. This matrix is named COVID Business Matrix (known as CoBuM hereafter). This matrix is designed to emphasize the unprecedented significant impact brought in by COVID-19 which is one of the most significant catastrophes with unimaginable impact on businesses and organizations across the world. The following section will provide an overview of these pillars.

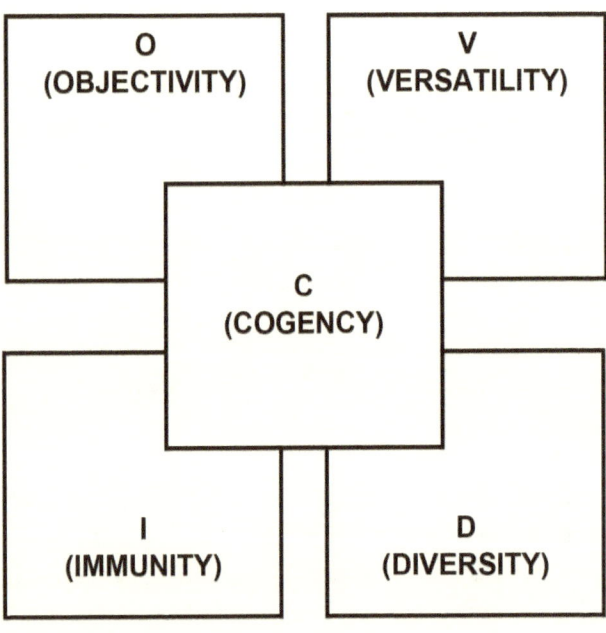

Figure 7.1 COVID Business Matrix

7.3.1 Cogency (C)

An organization is well-positioned to manage its contingencies when it is cogent, a quality of being clear, logical, and convincing with lucidity. Cogency refers to the ability of organizations to support their decisions with sufficient (logical) evidence to defend themselves against challenges coming from the environment within which it operates. This requires that ostensive references are made to provide a valid ground for efficient decision-making. This suggests that four dimensions can be considered for cogent decision-making in organizations to ensure their long-term sustainability: objectivity, versatility, immunity, and diversity.

Objectivity is concerned with the ability to maintain a realistic perspective while minimizing personal prejudices. It involves logical reasoning on how a decisive judgment regarding a state of affairs is made is being made objectively with adequate information from internal and external environments. Hence, evidence for decision-making must be clear, relevant, reasonable, and non-contradictory in their application of predicates, or they must adequately support the premises from a logical point of view to be considered logical. This also involves predictions and projections of diverse business scenarios through formal logic of deductive and inductive reasoning and the resulting strategic moves to cope with the contingencies. It is essential to note that links between premises and conclusions are very objective and provide a more informed strategic direction for the organization.

An ability to adapt or be adapted to many different business environment possibilities explains the second dimension within organizational cogency which is versatility. To be considered versatile, cogent decisions should incorporate versatility across the organizations that promote critical decision-making. A versatile organization is tuned to respond to challenges and is well prepared to rebuttal these challenges quickly without the coercion of force or time pressure. The versatility dimension, therefore, idealizes various business conditions and provides an opportunity for the organizations to be ready at all times for changing market dynamics.

Immunity, the third dimension within organizational cogency concerned with the strength of "organizational antibodies" in anticipating and addressing shocks as they come. The strength of the "antibody" depends on the degree of objectivity and also versatility in making decisive judgments while catering to the versatile needs of a continuously changing business environment. In other words, cogency in the organizations is not achieved not only through formal inductive and deductive (logical) reasoning but also through immunity of the organizations represented in the strength of the decisions asserting that competence to understand a business environment from a present and future state allows one making the judgment to be in a position to cast such a judgment.

The final dimension of diversity is associated with the degree of dissimilarity within the organization that stands out as a strength for long-term sustainability. This dimension focuses on how the organizations are strategizing the diversity in the organization for the best benefits of its long-term growth. Although a greater degree of diversity can be very challenging, the ability of the organizations to capitalize on it by understanding its uniqueness defines their long-term plan for performance as well as sustainability. The diversity dimension, therefore, acts as a means to scrutinize the conception and execution of a sustainable business strategy by creating the strategic fit between diversity and organizational strategies. A premise can therefore evoke that diversity conditions this need to be considered as essential to not undermine the cogency of the decision-making in the organizations.

This initial discussion suggests that all of these dimensions are very important for organizations. These dimensions are highly interrelated and need to be seen holistically by the organization while making decisions as there are many more upheavals that the organization will face in the future. The next section will explain each of these dimensions in more detail.

7.3.2 Objectivity (O)

The capacity to preserve a realistic viewpoint and minimize personal biases is referred to as objectivity. Organizations that follow objectivity rely on factual information in making scenario-specific decisions. Various biases from the organizational citizens such as previous experiences, and personal interests may influence the objectivity. However, a choice that is made objectively is not impacted by personal sentiments, viewpoints, interests, or prejudices. Rather, it takes into account only verifiable facts as well as the interests of all parties.

Objective descriptions are an important part of a competent decision-making process in decision science. Most crucially and realistically, objective description necessitates the employment of appropriate instruments and competence, as well as the appropriate resources. In this situation, judgment replaces, or more accurately, complements, objective description. Therefore, objectivity ensures adherence to the values of the organization with the ultimate aim of maximizing benefit and minimizing loss. In cases where there are conflicts or competing priorities, the organization must find an acceptable solution.

Regardless of viewpoint, objectivity in decision-making must be based purely on facts, data, and analysis that can be independently verified with a variety of perspectives agreed by rational and informed people.

7.3.3 Versatility (V)

Recent debates on organizational performance have stressed increasing complexity and a faster rate of change, and have called for new business models to deal with the paradoxes and difficulties that these factors create. On the surface, reacting to an unknown economic shock may be seen as overly confident and all-knowing by the citizens of the organizations. However, little do we acknowledge that business is just like gambling? In reality, all organizations are cautious, unsure, and puzzled, particularly when it comes to making quick judgments. So, how do the organizations keep their businesses sustainable? Their capacity to recognize and fix issues quickly is the key.

Addressing and overcoming business models which are inflexible as well as unresponsive to change is now becoming a major focus area the organizations. In this vein, organizations are striving to create dynamic and versatile organizational settings. However, the question is what is it that makes an organization stand out as a dynamic and versatile organization? When the operational environment changes, organizations should be able to swiftly reorganize their resources to successfully offer products or services that satisfy market needs by reacting to market dynamics. This requires realignment of the versatile leadership and operational process exemplified through different business models are developed for various products and services offered by the organization in meeting the diversified needs and wants of diverse customers from multiple market segments. This is one of the most important messages presented by the current catastrophe faced by organizations across the globe.

7.3.4 Immunity (I)

There are lessons to be learned from the health crisis for today's businesses in terms of building the immunities they'll need to be protected from future disruptive catastrophes. This is because only immune organizations' are well-positioned to withstand disruptions of any magnitude. In order to develop an immunity that can withstand future shocks, organizations are required to think far and beyond their existing boundaries so that they can overcome future disruptions. This immunity can be developed through various mechanisms including versatile business models supported by flexible organizational designs and enhancement and investments in technology.

It is undeniable that a "full immunity" may not be achieved by organizations. However, when the organizations are made to face the next major disruption, it may help the organizations get back on their feet much faster although it may not avoid a total commercial interruption. Bindra (2020) in Hindustan Times recommended several "antibodies" that an organization can develop. Firstly, organizations should opt for decentralization of work. This is because disruptions are managed well when the work structure is decentralized.

Secondly, the transformation of the business model that fits the needs of the digital world. It may not be possible for all organizations to transform into digitalized business models. However, restructuring the organization to be versatile requires a minimum level of digitalization. Organizations with conventional business models are no longer capable of coping with fast-changing market dynamics. Thirdly, it is recommended to develop a partnership ecosystem that complements their business models acknowledging resource scarcity is an unavoidable challenge in pursuing transformation. Fourthly, the organization's focus needed to be shifted towards automation opportunities and possibilities. This move does not only increases productivity but also helps in cost optimization in the long run. A company's immune system can be strengthened by immunizing itself against automation.

Fifthly, organizations must quickly reimagine the customer journeys. The Covid-19 cataclysmic event has made a tremendous change to consumer behaviors, their lifestyle, and the future of the consumer market. For any firm, this means adjusting their business for this new customer experience and future-proofing themselves. Finally, immunity can be developed only with changes in mindsets and organizational cultural transformation. It is necessary to produce the most powerful "antibody" of mindset and cultural transformation before developing any of the others. So much simpler to construct the others once they've been developed and internalized, resulting in high levels of organizational immunity.

7.3.5 Diversity (D)

Diversity is one of an organization's greatest assets. In today's extremely competitive global marketplace, diversity is essential to success although there are claims that diversity is a topic that corporate executives talk about, they do not practice it. Hence, it's apparent that diversity needs a facelift. Organizations need a business model that completely embraces diversity as a growth catalyst for businesses. The benefits of diversity in business are numerous, including the availability of talent, the enhancement of interpersonal creativity, the avoidance of risk, and the attractiveness to a worldwide consumer base.

More importantly, organizational diversity allows one to better serve the varied clientele. Because diversity may lead to better decision-making, better problem-solving, and higher creativity and invention - all of which can lead to superior product creation as well as more effective marketing to diverse sorts of clients - the commercial case for diversity is driven by this belief. Incorporating diversity into the organization increases innovation and creativity, as well as the company's adaptability and fast decision-making. Besides, through a broader and more complete perspective, diversity fosters distinctive thinking and better decision-making.

To seize opportunities and avoid external dangers, an organization needs to be nimble by capitalizing the diversity. This is based on a basic premise. Innovative thinking encourages organizations to think outside of the box, employing a variety of viewpoints to come up with fresh and distinctive findings, which is inherent in the process of staying sustainable despite a fast-changing environment. However, mismanagement poses a threat to diversity in the organization, despite its obvious benefits. Despite the drawbacks, when it comes to global business success, an organization's ability to effectively manage diversity will decide whether you succeed or fail in the long term.

7.4 RESPONSE STRATEGIES

It became apparent as the coronavirus and the disease became widespread that the organizations needed to take a long-term view of the existing situation and analyze prospects. In the wake of a frenetic period, organizations are finally forced to rethink their business models to seize opportunities presented by the environment. Some of the best possibilities exist for organizations that are flexible enough to reconfigure their existing business models. Four fundamentals are products and services, channels, infrastructure, and skills sets that have been identified to align organizational business models with evolving market developments depending on the quadrant they fit as discussed in chapter one, namely Preserve, Renew, Revive, and Exit. While imagining how a rebuilt world would appear, the following scenarios came into focus.

Table 7.1 Response Strategies

	Preserve	Renew	Revive	Exit
Agility	High	Low	High	Low
Resilience	High	High	Low	Low
Response Strategies				
Product and Services	Maintain	Adapt/Change	Maintain	Adapt/Change
Channel	Maintain	Maintain	Adapt/Change	Adapt/Change
Infrastructure	Maintain	Adapt/Change	Maintain	Adapt/Change
Skills	Maintain	Maintain	Adapt/Change	Adapt/Change

7.4.1 Preserve Strategy
Same Products and Services, Same Channel, Same Infrastructure, Same Skill

Organizations that fit within the Preserve strategy are the ones that have considered Cogency, Objectivity, Versatility, Immunity, and Diversity while deciding their business models. This indicates an optimistic and ideal state of an organization. It means, the organizations have developed a very adaptive business model sooner than expected and ahead of potential catastrophes. In this scenario, the disruptions to the business are managed well by adapting themselves quickly to the changing customer and market dynamics as a result of coordinated decision-making from the very beginning.

More specifically, the organizations' existing products and services, channels, infrastructure, and skills sets remain valid and reliable to overcome the disruptions. The characteristics and types of products and services are well-thought and it has taken into consideration the future needs of the consumer and markets. The channels used to communicate about the organizational offerings are also very futuristic in that it has the richness of information, reachability to the diversified customer segments, and established a strong affiliation with the present and potential customers. The infrastructure is up-to-date following the trends in the industry and able to do customization from time to time to capture and deliver values to the customer segments. In performing these activities, the existing skill sets are not only valuable but also valid, reliable, and in line with the current demands.

Ultimately, it is not easy to attain an ideal presence as discussed above. However, organizations are still presented with every opportunity to come closer to this ideal state by capitalizing on industry developments. These types of organizations tend to be first movers instead of being laggards. Although the disruption may create shocks to the existing business model, the time to return to normal operations will be shorter than expected. Organizations with such characteristics are portrayed by a higher level of resilience and agility.

7.4.2 Renew Strategy
Different Products and Services, Same Channel, Different Infrastructure, Different Skill

The sudden shock created by COVID-19 has shown a great impact on the demand and supply of products and services. Many products or services have witnessed dampening demand. This as a result has reduced capacity utilization and organizational infrastructures have become unused. Many industries stay stagnant without improvement. While the market for certain items and services has decreased, demand for others is robust and even increasing. Some businesses are capitalizing on this trend by repurposing current infrastructure to manufacture new goods or provide new sorts of services.

This reflects the renew response strategy where organizations attempt to venture into different products and services using the same channel. However, the organizations will require different infrastructure and different skill sets to be successful. When an organizational plan is developed to remedy failing performance, it is referred to as a renewal strategy. This sort of strategy assists an organization in stabilizing operations, revitalizing organizational resources and competencies, and repositioning itself to compete.

When an organization is functioning in a difficult environment, a renewal approach to the strategy may revitalize its energy and competitiveness. When conditions are so challenging that the existing manner of conducting business cannot be sustained, shifting course to save and free up resources and then later redirecting toward growth is the only way to not just survive, but eventually, thrive again.

Organizations following renew response strategy are portrayed with a higher level of resilience and a lower level of agility.

They will attempt to develop a higher level of versatility to accommodate the new change of course. Its new direction should be very objective by considering the disruptions created by sudden shocks to create stronger immunity to face future calamities. The organization should recognize and respond to the worsening environment to overcome immediate hurdles to financial sustainability or perhaps existence. This will support the next stage of the renewal journey.

7.4.3 Revive Strategy
Same Products and Services, Different Channel, Same Infrastructure, Different Skill

Offering the same (or comparable) products and services via the different and available channels is one proactive business response strategy to COVID-19. One potential strategy may include the digitalization of physical products or, in the case of services, through technology-mediated channels. This is best known as a revive response strategy. Organizations with such characteristics are portrayed by a higher level of agility and a lower level of resilience.

When organizations are well-positioned to learn from the past and add value to the present, revive response strategy may become an immediate option for financial sustainability and business continuity protecting the core business, and being ready for the future. Adoption of this strategy requires the deployment of aggressive short-term strategies by taking existing products or services to the market through technology-mediated platforms. This strategy needs people to be assertive with required competencies so that they are ready to anticipate the future.

In this vein, organizations pursuing revive strategy follows the same products and services, different channel, same infrastructure, but different skills structure. In this structure, organizations will retain only the relevant for their immediate survival by harnessing digital technologies to sustain and potentially create additional revenue streams.

All pillars described in COVID Business Matrix are also applicable to the organization adopting a revive response strategy. However, the main focus of the organization will be on the diversity of channels to reach a larger market with its existing products and services to enhance its immunity to business disruptions.

7.4.4 Exit Strategy
Different Products and Services, Different Channel, Different Infrastructure, Different Skill

An exit strategy can be a difficult decision to make when an organization becomes no longer profitable. The goal of an exit strategy is to reduce losses or maximize personal profit. An organization will be forced to adopt an exit response strategy when its current products and services, its channels, infrastructure, and skills sets are no longer accommodating the changes in market dynamics as a result of sudden shocks.

Such a situation indicates that the organization failed to ensure cogency, objectivity, versatility, immunity, and also diversity of its business and operations. Organizations with such characteristics are portrayed with a lower level of resilience and agility. When the organizations are struggling to meet the changing preferences of the market and the industry is making a shift towards a new way of doing business, the existing strategy becomes the only option to be adopted.

While exit strategy can be a difficult decision, the organization usually will be presented with no option but to exit the market to avoid further losses. The organization needs to quickly augment its products and services, channel, infrastructure, and skillsets in line with changing preferences if the organization intends to stay in the market and industry. However, is easier said than done and often requires extensive effort, time, and resources to bridge such gaps.

7.5 CONCLUSION

The COVID-19 pandemic has sparked a shift in how organizations should approach their business model in the future as they cope with day-to-day operations. This issue has prompted organizations to change the way they operate, manage their workforce, and respond to consumer and employee needs. We anticipate that the business world will appear very different post-COVID-19 although the outlook for immediate recovery still looks gloomy.

Hence, the overall aim of the book has been to investigate the impacts of COVID-19 on businesses, the plausible organizational scenarios, and also potential remedial strategies. The discussion is grounded in both relevant literature and the practical experiences of the authors. This is just an early descriptive contribution. However, our contribution is envisaged to help organizations to position themselves and establish a realistic recovery path while working on CoBuM to ensure their long-term sustainability considering that uneven recovery ensues and similar future anomalies are unavoidable.

It is important to note that the plausible organizational scenarios and corresponding response strategies may vary for the organizations depending on their industries, relevant markets, geographical footprints, workforces competencies and diversities, and more. Nevertheless, we believe our contribution provides a valuable insight for organizations to establish a flexible business framework characterized by resilience and agility for long-term performance and growth in the future.

Despite the current state of the organizations, we opined that organizations must first determine the scope of their goal of immediate recovery and how it connects to their entire strategy for long-term sustainability. This will enable the management of the organization to reshape its efforts and fix attainable targets that can be communicated across the organization to create the alignment across functions for recovery as well as the creation of versatility, immunity, and diversity in the future business strategies for the business to remain cogent.

ACKNOWLEDGEMENT

Writing a book is harder than I thought and more rewarding than I could have ever imagined. None of this would have been possible without motivation and encouragement from my family, friends, and everyone who was involved directly or indirectly by contributing ideas and perspectives. Finally, my sincere appreciation to all those who have been a part of my getting there.

REFERENCES

Bindra, J. (2020). 'Immune organizations' can withstand disruptions. Hindustan Times. Retrieved from https://www.hindustantimes.com/analysis/immune-organisations-can-withstand-disruptions/story-F7ZJ3diop4K2YWB4pJ3pzI.html on 12 September 2021.